The Ultimate Diet Tool Kit

Ohio Distinctive Software Guide to Diet and Nutrition

Stanford Apseloff and Glen Apseloff, M.D.

The Ultimate Diet Tool Kit

Ohio Distinctive Software Guide to
Diet and Nutrition

Stanford Apseloff and Glen Apseloff, M.D.

OHIO DISTINCTIVE SOFTWARE, INC.
Columbus, Ohio 1994

There are many people who have made this book possible, and while they expect no acknowledgement for their contributions, they deserve much more than this brief mention. Mom and Dad, Roy and Lynn, thank you for the lifetime of encouragement and support. Sheri Schwarz, thank you for your help and loyalty that began long before this book. Ohio Distinctive Software operations and marketing, including the exceptionally dedicated Sherie Garesche and the resourceful Erich Speer, and highly-professional production staff Joseph Boone, Mary Ellen Cerny, Mary Ellen Krecic, Andrew Collins and Bill Price, thank you. And last but not least, for her fastidious editing and the creation of an index, thank you Diane Chambers.

Published by Ohio Distinctive Software, Inc., 4588 Kenny Rd., Columbus OH 43220.

Printed in the United States of America.

97 8 7 6 5 4

ISBN: 0-9647934-0-7

Contents

This book is based on four best-selling nutrition software products of Ohio Distinctive Software: *Executive Diet Helper*, *Menu Planner*, *Weight Loss Planner*, and *Food Label Analyzer*.

The information in this book is designed to supplement your knowledge of diet and nutrition. However, because of the great volume of information and the ever-changing nature of packaged and processed goods, and the inherent complexity of the algorithms used to create the information contained herein, we cannot guarantee the complete accuracy of all the material. Also, because individual needs vary greatly, it is extremely important that before undertaking any change in diet, nutrition or exercise, you seek professional advice from your physician or dietitian.

INTRODUCTION

This diet book is different from all the others. It is not a miracle weight-loss plan, nor is it a technical manual. It is simply the ultimate diet tool kit.

With the tools provided in this book, you will be able to better understand, monitor and control your diet. Whether your goal is to lose weight, limit consumption of fat, or simply gain a better understanding of what you eat, the tools in this book will help. If you think it is time to take control of your diet, then this book is for you.

This book begins with a brief discussion of diet and exercise guidelines. The chapters that follow contain the tools you need to select and/or prepare healthful foods. Specifically, the chapter on menu plans contains menus for different calorie levels and provides a broad selection of foods within each menu plan. It encourages selection of low-fat foods and provides a relatively balanced diet at any of the calorie levels listed. It is designed to maximize ease of use and choice in food selection. With the menu plans in this book, you will be able to control your caloric intake without restricting yourself to foods you do not like.

The chapter of exercise graphs is a set of two tools. The first enables you to determine the number of calories expended during exercise, while the second enables you to determine the weight loss attributable to exercise.

The chapter on shoppers' guidelines provides a tool for selecting foods that meet your dietary criteria. Specifically, the guidelines are a quick and easy reference for determining whether foods have more than a specified percentage of calories derived from fat. Although government regulations do require food companies to provide some nutritional information on food product labels, the information on fat is a % Daily Value based on 2000 Calories (rather than being based on the calories in a single serving of the food). There is no requirement that labels list the percentage of calories from fat. As a result, a food label may indicate a low percentage of fat, even if a food is 100% fat! (E.g., margarine has a % Daily Value for fat of only 22% even though it is 100% fat.) Our shoppers' guideline tool will enable you to make wise choices based on the guidelines you want.

The food analysis section of this book is a tool for selecting specific foods and specific methods of food preparation. This chapter lists the calories, carbohydrates, protein, fat and cholesterol in foods and provides suggestions on lower-calorie/lower-fat substitute choices. The foods are divided into seventeen categories and are listed in alphabetical order within each category for easy access. The information is a powerful tool for either analyzing or modifying an existing diet, in conjunction with the guidance provided by your physician or dietitian.

The chapter of nutrition tables lists the vitamin and mineral content of selected foods. It is a convenient tool for determining which foods you might choose if you wish to increase your consumption of certain vitamins or minerals. The foods at the top of some of these lists may surprise you.

Please note: you should discuss your personal nutritional needs and goals with your physician or dietitian to ensure proper use of this book. Do not undertake any change in diet or exercise without first consulting your physician or registered/licensed dietitian.

NUTRITION & EXERCISE GUIDELINES

NUTRITION GUIDELINES

General Information -- Fat, protein, carbohydrates and alcohol are the source of all calories in our diet. All types of fat contain roughly 9 calories per gram, more than twice as many calories as pure sugar! Protein and carbohydrates each contain approximately 4 calories per gram, while alcohol has approximately 7 calories per gram. A gain (or loss) in consumption of 3500 calories results in a gain (or loss) of approximately 1 pound of body weight. Therefore, in order to lose 1 pound in 1 week, your body must, each day, burn 500 calories more than you consume as food. Water contains no calories, so drinking it does not cause any increase in body fat, and a decrease in consumption of water does not aid in meaningful weight loss.

Fat and Cholesterol -- Fat is the most densely caloric substance, more than twice as caloric as sugar. One ounce of fat contains approximately 250 calories! To avoid fat, therefore, is to avoid calories. Many people find that if they reduce the amount of fat in their diet, they are still able to eat a satisfying quantity of food while dieting to lose weight. For example, a complete meal consisting of two skinless, grilled chicken sandwiches, a baked potato and green beans contains fewer calories than one hamburger and an order of French fries. (See the Food Analysis chapter of this book.) In addition to the fact that a diet high in fat is a diet high in calories, the American Cancer Society cautions that a high-fat diet may increase the risk of developing breast, colon or prostate cancer.

It is important to note that olive oil, corn oil or any other type of oil is 100% fat. If you are trying to reduce your consumption of fat, switching from lard to olive oil won't help. Again, see the Food Analysis chapter of this book.

Cholesterol is a close relative of fat. It is found only in animal products. Vegetable oils contain no cholesterol, yet 100% of their calories comes from fat. Therefore, avoiding cholesterol will not ensure that you have a low-fat diet. The tools in this book, however, will enable you to monitor and reduce intake of fat and cholesterol.

The Food and Nutrition Board of the National Research Council has determined that the Recommended Dietary Allowance of fat is not more than 30% of calories and the Recommended Dietary Allowance of cholesterol is not more than 300 mg per day.

Protein -- The Recommended Dietary Allowance of protein for adult males and females ranges from 46 grams to 65 grams. These figures are based on 0.75 grams of protein per kg (2.2 lbs.) of body weight, plus an additional 10 grams of protein for women who are pregnant, an additional 15 grams for women in the first 6 months of lactation, dropping to 12 additional grams for the second 6 months of lactation.

Alcohol -- Alcohol contains 7 calories per gram. A 1.5-ounce shot of 100-proof vodka, gin or rum (50% alcohol) contains about 150 calories! If you drink daily on a social basis, you may be surprised to find that 10% or more of your daily calories comes from alcohol. Many moderate social drinkers have been able to lose a considerable amount of weight simply by abstaining from alcohol. The American Heart Association recommends a maximum of 1 to 2 ounces of alcohol per day. In addition, the American Cancer Society recommends moderation and cautions that heavy drinkers are more likely to develop some types of cancer.

Sugar -- Although sugar does contain fewer calories than either fat or alcohol, it too should be consumed in moderation. Foods that are high in added sugar are often high in fat as well (e.g., candy bars). Also, sugar is used in processed foods in much greater volumes than most people are aware. For example, one 12-ounce soft drink contains approximately 9 teaspoons of sugar!

Food Selection -- The human body requires a vast array of vitamins, minerals, amino acids (the building blocks of protein) and other nutrients. Elimination of entire food groups from your diet, or even concentration on a few types of food to the exclusion of others, risks depriving your body of essential nourishment. If the diet you are contemplating does not allow for consumption of a wide variety of foods, be sure to consult your health professional regarding potential risks. Again please note: before starting any diet, consult your physician or registered/licensed dietitian.

EXERCISE GUIDELINES

Benefits of Regular Exercise -- While the advantages of exercising regularly may vary from person to person, you may reasonably expect to experience some or all of the following benefits:

1. Weight loss/weight control
2. Increased muscle-tone
3. Increased endurance
4. Increased capacity for physical work
5. Reduced risk of heart attack
6. Improved self-confidence

In addition, exercise can be an important factor in reducing stress, fatigue, insomnia, depression and anxiety.

Tips for Exercise Program Development -- Experts brought together by the U.S. Centers for Disease Control and Prevention and the American College of Sports Medicine, in cooperation with the President's Council on Physical Fitness and Sports, recommend that every American adult accumulate 30 minutes or more of moderate-intensity physical activity over the course of most days of the week. This 30 minutes may come from daily activities such as walking, raking leaves, gardening, etc., or it may come from planned exercise or recreation.

For those individuals who wish to set up an exercise program, the following advice may be useful: First, consult your physician before starting any type of exercise. Then, begin slowly. Your particular condition and needs will dictate how slowly you should begin and how rapidly you will be able to progress. Pain, nausea, lightheadedness, and other unusual sensations are warning signs; stop exercising and consult your physician. To obtain the maximum cardiovascular benefit and burn the greatest number of calories, select exercises that have relatively continuous, uninterrupted activity, such as running, walking, cycling, rowing, swimming, etc. (See Exercise Graphs chapter.) The American Heart Association recommends that your goal should be to exercise at least 20 to 30 minutes, three times per week or more, at a "moderate" level. "Moderate" means that the exercise raises your heart rate to a range of 60% to 75% of its "maximum". ("Maximum" heart rate is usually 220 minus your age.) Please refer to the following table:

Age	Exercise Heart-Rate Goal*	Avg. Maximum**
20	120-150 beats per minute	200
25	117-146 beats per minute	195
30	114-142 beats per minute	190
35	111-138 beats per minute	185
40	108-135 beats per minute	180
45	105-131 beats per minute	175
50	102-127 beats per minute	170
55	99-123 beats per minute	165
60	96-120 beats per minute	160
65	93-116 beats per minute	155
70	90-113 beats per minute	150

* Immediately after exercising, count your pulse for 15 seconds and multiply by 4 to see if you exercised in the range of your heart-rate goal.

* * Do not try to attain maximum heart rate!

WARNING:

1. Excessive exercise may cause joint or muscle injuries.
2. Exercise in extreme weather can be dangerous.
3. Pain during moderate exercise is not normal.

Warm up before exercising, and cool down afterwards. (Consult a professional for advice about different types of stretching and calisthenics.)

MENU PLANS

INTRODUCTION

The following menu plans are a tool for maintaining your desired daily calorie level. These menu plans are more than just lists of food; instead of dictating what you must eat and avoid, they provide you with knowledge and choice. On a calorie-restricted diet, there is clearly a trade-off between caloric density and serving size. Some diet plans force the decision upon you by requiring that you eat specific foods in specific quantities. With our menu plans, you make the decisions. If you are not very hungry but you have a craving for a certain food, our menu plans will accommodate your desire. If you are very hungry and wish to eat a large quantity of food, our menu plans enable that as well.

Our menu plans contain foods that are divided into three categories: calorie light, calorie moderate and calorie dense. In most cases these three food categories represent low-fat, moderate-fat and high-fat foods. You will note that on a diet consisting of primarily calorie-dense foods, it is virtually impossible to avoid weight gain without being hungry. With the calorie-light foods, however, you should be able to eat a quantity of food sufficient to keep you from feeling hungry, regardless of which plan you select. The menu plans, therefore, will guide you toward low-fat/low-calorie food selections. To obtain information on the fat content of specific foods, refer to the Food Analysis chapter of this book.

The menu plans in this chapter represent a range of daily calorie levels from 1200 to 2000. There are two menu plans for each calorie level to ensure that you have a wide range of choices in the foods you select.

Your physician or dietitian can tell you which daily calorie level is best for you. If your needs fall outside the range of our menu plans, you can still use our plans by simply taking a fraction or a multiple of the values of the plans listed. For example, to follow a menu plan for 2400 calories per day, simply use the 1200-calorie-per-day menu plan and double all the quantities.

Please note that regardless of which menu plan you use, there will be some variation in the actual number of calories you consume because there is some variation in the brands of foods and the proportion of ingredients. Where appropriate, we have attempted to minimize some of these variations by classifying foods with obvious differences in different categories (e.g., sandwiches with mayonnaise versus sandwiches without mayonnaise). Again, if you have questions about the caloric content of specific foods on any of the plans, refer to the Food Analysis chapter of this book.

For the menu plans in this book, in addition to consuming the foods listed, you may drink as much water, seltzer, diet soda, black coffee and unsweetened tea as you desire without adding any calories to your diet. Also keep in mind that while herbs and spices add almost no calories to your diet, mustard, relish and ketchup add some, while mayonnaise, butter and oils add a lot. Celery, cucumbers, lettuce and radishes are particularly low in calories, which means that extra amounts of these can be consumed without significantly raising your daily caloric intake.

With our menu plans you will find that some calorie-light foods have serving sizes that are unusually large. This means that you may consume as much of these foods as you desire, not that you are required to eat that amount.

You may wish to use a kitchen food scale to obtain an accurate reading of the weight of your food. Or, for packaged foods, there is often information on the packaging that enables you to estimate the weight of servings with reasonable accuracy. Finally, if you do not have a kitchen scale and there is no other serving-size information available, use the list (on the next page) of approximate weights of foods in common units.

Again, please note that everyone's dietary needs are different, and you should consult your physician or dietitian to determine which menu plan is best for you.

APPROXIMATE WEIGHT OF FOOD IN COMMON UNITS

1. Beverages, soup, gravy, syrup, salad dressing and other liquid:
   1 cup weighs approximately 8 ounces.
   1 tablespoon weighs approximately 0.5 ounce.
2. Bread, crackers, nuts and popcorn:
   1 slice of bread weighs approximately 1 ounce.
   1 bagel weighs approximately 2 ounces.
   8 Ritz crackers weigh approximately 1 ounce.
   30 Virginia peanuts, shelled, weigh approximately 1 ounce.
   18 medium-size cashews weigh approximately 1 ounce.
   1 cup of popped popcorn weighs approximately 1/4 ounce.
3. Cereal:
   1 bowl of corn flakes (1 cup) weighs approximately 1 ounce.
   1 bowl of raisin bran (1 cup) weighs approximately 2 ounces.
   1 bowl hot cereal (e.g., 1 cup oatmeal) weighs approximately 8 oz.
4. Dessert:
   1 piece of cake (3x3x2 inches) weighs approximately 3 ounces.
   1 piece of pie (3.5 inch sector, 1/8 total pie) weighs approx. 4 oz.
   3 Oreo cookies weigh approximately 1 ounce.
   1 cup of ice cream weighs approximately 5 ounces.
5. Eggs and omelets:
   1 large egg weighs approximately 2 ounces.
   1 three-egg omelet weighs approximately 8 ounces.
6. Fruit and vegetables:
   1 apple, orange, peach or pear weighs approximately 5 ounces.
   1 cup of mixed vegetables weighs approximately 6.5 ounces.
7. Meat:
   4 slices of cooked bacon weigh approximately 1 ounce.
   1 slice of lunch meat weighs approximately 1 ounce.
   1 hot dog weighs approximately 1.6 ounces.
8. Pizza:
   1 pie (12 inch diameter) weighs approximately 20 ounces.
9. Pasta:
   1 cup weighs approximately 5 ounces.
10. Rice:
    1 cup weighs approximately 6 ounces.
11. Sandwiches:
    1 average homemade sandwich weighs approximately 6 ounces.
    1 fast-food small hamburger weighs approximately 4 ounces.
    1 Quarter Pounder with cheese weighs approximately 6.5 ounces.

SUMMARY OF MENU PLANS

DAILY MENU PLAN #1 -- 1200 CALORIES

Breakfast: Breakfast meat, egg dish, juice
Lunch: Meat, soup, fruit, milk product
Dinner: Salad, entree, rice/potato, vegetables, dessert

DAILY MENU PLAN #2 -- 1200 CALORIES

Breakfast: Breakfast bread, cereal, fruit
Lunch: Sandwich, salad, juice, cheese/yogurt
Dinner: Salad, meat, bread, vegetables, dessert

DAILY MENU PLAN #3 -- 1400 CALORIES

Breakfast: Breakfast meat, egg dish, juice
Lunch: Meat, soup, fruit, milk product
Dinner: Salad, entree, rice/potato, vegetables, dessert

DAILY MENU PLAN #4 -- 1400 CALORIES

Breakfast: Breakfast bread, cereal, fruit
Lunch: Sandwich, salad, juice, cheese/yogurt
Dinner: Salad, meat, bread, vegetables, dessert

DAILY MENU PLAN #5 -- 1600 CALORIES

Breakfast: Breakfast meat, egg dish, juice
Lunch: Meat, soup, fruit, milk product
Dinner: Salad, entree, rice/potato, vegetables, dessert

DAILY MENU PLAN #6 -- 1600 CALORIES

Breakfast: Breakfast bread, cereal, fruit
Lunch: Sandwich, salad, juice, cheese/yogurt
Dinner: Salad, meat, bread, vegetables, dessert

DAILY MENU PLAN #7 -- 1800 CALORIES

Breakfast: Breakfast meat, egg dish, juice
Lunch: Meat, soup, fruit, milk product
Dinner: Salad, entree, rice/potato, vegetables, dessert

DAILY MENU PLAN #8 -- 1800 CALORIES

Breakfast: Breakfast bread, cereal, fruit
Lunch: Sandwich, salad, juice, cheese/yogurt
Dinner: Salad, meat, bread, vegetables, dessert

DAILY MENU PLAN #9 -- 2000 CALORIES

Breakfast: Breakfast meat, egg dish, juice
Lunch: Meat, soup, fruit, milk product
Dinner: Salad, entree, rice/potato, vegetables, dessert

DAILY MENU PLAN #10 -- 2000 CALORIES

Breakfast: Breakfast bread, cereal, fruit
Lunch: Sandwich, salad, juice, cheese/yogurt
Dinner: Salad, meat, bread, vegetables, dessert

MENU PLAN EXCHANGES

You may mix and match parts of menu plans if you adhere to the following guidelines:

1. Mix and match only with menu plans that have identical calorie levels (e.g., Menu Plans #1 and #2, but not Plans #1 and #4).
2. Use the serving sizes that are assigned to the particular foods. For example, you may substitute 4 ounces of "garden salad, no dressing" for an unlimited amount of "bouillon".
3. You may exchange entire meals from one menu plan to another (e.g., exchange dinner in Menu Plan #2 for dinner in Plan #1).
4. You may exchange specific foods selections as long as the foods occupy the same position in the Menu Plans. For example, for Menu Plan #1 thc second food selection "egg dishes" may be exchanged for the Plan #2 second food selection "cereals".
5. You may eat a combination of foods within a category as long as they are in the same classification of calorie light, moderate or dense. For example, instead of eating 8 ounces of asparagus for Menu Plan #1 dinner, you may choose to eat 4 ounces of asparagus and 4 ounces of broccoli.

DAILY MENU PLAN #1 -- 1200 CALORIES

BREAKFAST -- Choose 1 item from each section (i.e., choose 1 breakfast meat, 1 egg dish, and 1 juice). Select mostly "Light" foods.

Calorie Light	Calorie Moderate	Calorie Dense
(2.5 ounces)	(2.5 ounces)	(1.5 ounce)
Canadian bacon	Headcheese	Bacon (1.0 ounce)
Corned/roast beef hash	Regular ham	Blood sausage
Honey roll sausage, beef	Scrapple	Brown & serve sausage
Lean ham		Ham patties
New Eng. brand sausage		Other pork/beef sausage
Souse		Sirloin steak
(10.0 ounces)	(3.0 ounces)	(2.0 ounces)
Egg beaters	Fried eggs	Deviled eggs
Egg beater/cheese(4.0 oz)	Hard-boiled eggs	Egg yolks (1.5 ounces)
Egg whites	Omelets (2.5 ounces)	Quiche
	Other eggs	
	Poached eggs	
	Scrambled eggs	
	Soft-boiled eggs	
(4.0 ounces)	(3.0 ounces)	(0.5 ounce)
Apple cider	Apricot nectar	Coconut milk
Apple juice	Cranberry juice	
Blackberry juice	Cran-apple juice	
Grapefruit juice	Cran-apricot juice	
Grapefruit juice, sweetnd	Cran-grape juice	
Orange juice	Grape juice	
Orange-grapefruit juice	Orange-apricot juice	
Tangerine juice	Papaya nectar	
Tangelo juice	Passion fruit juice	
Tomato juice (8.0 ounces)	Peach or pear nectar	
	Pineapple juice	
	Pineapple-grapefrt juice	
	Pineapple-orange juice	
	Pine-orange-banana juice	
	Prune juice	

LUNCH -- Choose 1 item from each section. Select mostly "Light" foods.

Calorie Light	Calorie Moderate	Calorie Dense
(6.5 ounces)	(5.0 ounces)	(3.0 ounces)
Any 91% fat-free meat	Any 82% fat-free meat	All other lunch meat
Crab	Beef flank steak	All other pork
Fish canned in water	*Calf heart	Anything w/butter sauce
Lean ham	Lean lamb	Anything w/cream sauce
Lobster	*Liver	Anything with cheese
Other fish, not fried	Pork feet	Beef ribs
*Other organ meat	*Pork pancreas	Beef/pork tongue
Other seafood	Poultry, dark meat	Fried chicken/fried meat
Pork tenderloin, lean	Poultry with skin	Fried fish/fried seafood
Poultry, white w/gravy	Regular ham	Hamburger/meatloaf
Poultry, white w/o skin	Veal	Hot dog/sausage/kielbasa
Raw/steamed clams	Wild game	Other pork
Shrimp		Other steak/other beef
		Pork tail
*very high in cholesterol	*very high cholesterol	Poultry, dark w/skin
(5.5 ounces)	(3.5 ounces)	(2.5 ounces)
Bouillon (unlimited amt)	Soup, black bean	Soup, any chunky kind
Soup, beef mushroom	Soup, chicken dumpling	Soup, any made w/milk
Soup, beef noodle	Soup, cream of, w/water	Soup, bean w/bacon
Soup, chicken gumbo	Soup, pepper pot	Soup, bean w/franks
Soup, chicken noodle	Soup, tomato bisque	Soup, cheese
Soup, chicken vegetable	Soup, tomato with rice	Soup, chicken mushrm
Soup, chicken with rice		Soup, chili beef
Soup, Manh clam chowdr		Soup, N.E. clam chowdr
Soup, minestrone		Soup, pea green
Soup, mushrm w/barley		Soup, split pea w/ham
Soup, onion		Soup, tomato beef noodl
Soup, oyster stew w/watr		
Soup, Scotch broth		
Soup, tomato (w/water)		
Soup, turkey noodle		
Soup, turkey vegetable		
Soup, vegetable beef		
Soup, vegetarian vegetabl		

(4.0 ounces)	(2.5 ounces)	(0.5 ounce)
Fruit canned in juice	Bananas	Candied fruit
Fruit canned light syrup	Breadfruit	Coconut
Other fresh fruit	Crabapples	Dates
	Elderberries	Dried Fruit
	Fresh figs	Prunes
	Fruit canned hvy syrup	Raisins
	Passion fruit	
	Plantain	
	Sweetened fruit	

(9.0 ounces)	(5.0 ounces)	(3.0 ounces)
Cultured buttermilk	Chocolate milk	Eggnog
Low-fat milk	Coffee flavor milk	Hot cocoa made w/milk
Skim milk	Low-fat chocolate milk	Milk shake
	Whole goat milk	Whole sheep milk
	Whole milk	

DINNER -- Choose 1 item from each section. Select mostly "Light" foods.

Calorie Light	Calorie Moderate	Calorie Dense
(8.0 ounces)	(2.5 ounces)	(0.5 ounce)
Garden salad, no dressing	Salad with croutons	Any salad w/dressing
Salad with no-fat dressing	Salad with olives	Any salad w/mayonnaise
		Any salad with oil
		Chef salad/Caesar salad
(5.0 ounces)	(3.0 ounces)	(2.0 ounces)
Beef stew	Burritos	Cheese fondue
Casserole in tomato sauce	Chicken a la king	Chili con queso
Chili	Corned beef hash	Meatloaf
Diet entrees, except fried	Curry dishes with rice	Nachos
Pasta in tomato sauce	Enchiladas	Pasta in cream sauce
Shrimp creole	Macaroni and cheese	Pasta w/carbonara sauce
	Newburg dishes w/pasta	Stuffed potato skins
	Newburg dishes w/rice	Quiche
	Other casseroles	
	Other frozen entrees	
	Other pasta w/cheese	
	Other pasta w/meat	
	Pizza	
	Pot pies	
	Tacos	
	Tuna casserole	
(3.0 ounces)	(2.0 ounces)	(1.0 ounce)
Any rice/potato w/gravy	Any rice/potato w/butter	Any fried potatoes
Plain baked potato	Any rice/potato w/chees	Potato skins, baked/fried
Plain boiled potato	Baked potato, sour crm	
Plain brown rice	Beef flavored rice	
Plain white rice	Chicken flavored rice	
Scalloped potatoes	Chinese fried rice	
Spanish rice	Other flavored rice	

(8.0 ounces)	(4.0 ounces)	(2.0 ounces)
Asparagus	Acorn/butternut squash	Any deep fry veg(0.5 oz)
Bamboo shoots	Beets	Any veg w/butter, marg
Broccoli	Brussels sprouts	Any veg w/cheese sauce
Butterbur	Carrots	Arrowhead
Cauliflower	Hubbard/winter squash	Baked beans
Crookneck/scallop squash	Hyacinth beans	Broad beans
Eggplant	Kale	Corn/creamed corn
Rhubarb	Leeks	Green peas/cowpeas
Sauerkraut	Mixed vegetables	Kidney/pinto beans
Spaghetti/summer squash	Navy beans	Lima beans
Spinach	Okra	Parsnips
String beans	Onions	Pigeon peas
Fresh or stewed tomatoes	Rutabagas	Soybeans
Turnips	Shellie beans	Succotash
Zucchini	Winged beans	Sweet potatoes/yams

(4.0 ounces)	(1.5 ounce)	(0.5 ounce)
Fresh fruit	Frozen yogurt (2.5 oz)	Cake and pastry
Gelatin dessert	Fudgsicles	Candy and chocolate
Gelatin w/fruit	Ice milk	Cookies
Lo cal gelatin (unlimited)	Popsicles (2.5 ounces)	Ice cream/sundae (1.0 oz)
Lo cal popsicle (unlimit)	Pudding	Pie (1.0 ounce)
Lo cal pudding	Sherbert	

DAILY MENU PLAN #2 -- 1200 Calories

BREAKFAST -- Choose 1 item from each section (i.e., choose 1 breakfast bread product, 1 cereal, and 1 fruit). Select mostly "Light" foods.

Calorie Light	Calorie Moderate	Calorie Dense
(2.5 ounces)	(1.5 ounces)	(1.0 ounce)
French toast with syrup	Bagel with cream cheese	Biscuits with butter
Pancakes with syrup	Brown & serve rolls	Croissant
Plain bagel, any type	Coffee cake	Croissant with butter
Plain cornbread, homemd	English muffin w/butter	Danish pastry
Plain English muffins	Muffins, any type	Donuts, any type
Plain toast, low calorie	Pancakes w/butter,syrup	Matzo with butter
Toast w/low cal spread	Plain biscuits	
Waffles with syrup	Sweet rolls	
	Toast w/butter and jelly	
	Waffles w/butter, syrup	

Calorie Light	Calorie Moderate	Calorie Dense
(7.5 ounces)	(1.0 ounces)	(1.0 ounce)
Cream of wheat, cooked	*Bran cereals	*Granola-type cereals
Grits, cooked	*Flakes w/dried fruit	*Sugar-coated cereals
Malt-o-meal, cooked	*Other cereals	*High-sugar cereals
Maypo, cooked	*Plain flakes, any type	
Oatmeal, any type,cooked	*Wheat squares w/fruit	
Other hot cereal, cooked		
Ralston, cooked		
Wheatena, cooked	*Plus skim milk (4.0 oz)	*Plus skim milk (4.0 oz)

Calorie Light	Calorie Moderate	Calorie Dense
(3.5 ounces)	(2.0 ounces)	(0.5 ounce)
Fruit canned in juice	Bananas	Candied fruit
Fruit canned in lt syrup	Breadfruit	Coconut
Other fresh fruit	Crabapples	Dates
	Elderberries	Dried fruit
	Fresh figs	Prunes
	Fruit canned hvy syrup	Raisins
	Passion fruit	
	Plantain	
	Sweetened fruit	

LUNCH -- Choose 1 item from each section. Select mostly "Light" foods.

Calorie Light	Calorie Moderate	Calorie Dense
(5.0 ounces)	(4.0 ounces)	(3.5 ounces)
Sndwch,91% fat-free meat	Sndwch, 82-92% fat-free	Any croissant sandwich
Sandwich, grilled fish	Sandwich, regular ham	Any fried sandwich
Sandwich, grilled chicken		Any sandwich w/bacon
Sandwich, tuna (in water)		Any sandwich w/cheese
Sandwich, turkey		Any sandwich w/mayo
Sandwich, turkey breast		Burger/hot dog, all types
Sndwch, vegetarian(8.0oz)		Sandwich, meatball
		Sandwich, other meat
		Sndwch, p.b. &/or jelly
		Sandwich, submarine

Calorie Light	Calorie Moderate	Calorie Dense
(8.0 ounces)	(3.5 ounces)	(1.5 ounce)
Garden salad, no dressing	Salad with croutons	Any salad w/dressing
Salad with no-fat dressing	Salad with olives	Any salad w/mayonnaise
		Any salad with oil
		Chef salad/Caesar salad

Calorie Light	Calorie Moderate	Calorie Dense
(5.0 ounces)	(3.5 ounces)	(1.0 ounce)
Apple cider	Apricot nectar	Coconut milk
Apple juice	Cranberry juice	
Blackberry juice	Cran-apple juice	
Grapefruit juice	Cran-apricot juice	
Grapefruit juice, sweetnd	Cran-grape juice	
Orange juice	Grape juice	
Orange-grapefruit juice	Orange-apricot juice	
Tangerine juice	Papaya nectar	
Tangelo juice	Passion fruit juice	
Tomato juice (10.0 oz)	Peach nectar	
	Pear nectar	
	Pineapple juice	
	Pineapple-grapefrt juice	
	Pineapple-orange juice	
	Pine-orange-banana juice	
	Prune juice	

(4.5 ounces)	(1.5 ounces)	(1.0 ounces)
Cottage cheese, any type	Feta cheese	All other cheese
Lite ricotta	Neufchatel cheese	
Frozen yogurt	Part-skim mozzarella	
Yogurt, any type	Ricotta cheese	
	Skim mozzarella cheese	

DINNER -- Choose 1 item from each section. Select mostly "Light" foods.

Calorie Light	Calorie Moderate	Calorie Dense
(8.0 ounces)	(3.5 ounces)	(1.5 ounce)
Garden salad, no dressing	Salad with croutons	Any salad w/dressing
Salad with no-fat dressing	Salad with olives	Any salad w/mayonnaise
		Any salad with oil
		Chef salad/Caesar salad
(4.0 ounces)	(3.0 ounces)	(2.0 ounces)
Any 91% fat-free meat	Any 82% fat-free meat	All other lunch meat
Crab	Beef flank steak	All other pork
Fish canned in water	*Calf heart	Anything w/butter sauce
Lean ham	Lean lamb	Anything w/cream sauce
Lobster	*Liver	Anything with cheese
Other fish, not fried	Pork feet	Beef ribs
*Other organ meat	*Pork pancreas	Beef/pork tongue
Other seafood	Poultry, dark meat	Fried chicken/fried meat
Pork tenderloin, lean	Poultry with skin	Fried fish/fried seafood
Poultry, white w/gravy	Regular ham	Hamburger/meatloaf
Poultry, white w/o skin	Veal	Hot dog/sausage/kielbasa
Raw/steamed clams	Wild game	Other pork
Shrimp		Other steak/other beef
		Pork tail
*very high in cholesterol	*very high cholesterol	Poultry, dark w/skin
(1.0 ounces)	(0.5 ounce)	(0.5 ounce)
Plain bagels, any type	Bagels w/cream cheese	All other crackers
Cornbread	Bread/rolls with butter	All other nuts
Plain muffins, any type	Croissants	Cheetos/cheese curls
Plain bread/rolls	Honey-coated grahams	Chex snack mix
Roasted chestnuts	Matzo/bread sticks	Chips, any variety
	Oyster crackers	Microwave popcorn
	Plain air-pop popcorn	Popcorn, oil popped
	Plain graham crackers	Popcorn with butter
	Pretzels	Seeds, any type
	Soda crackers	
	Triscuit crackers	

(8.0 ounces)	(4.0 ounces)	(2.0 ounces)
Asparagus	Acorn/butternut squash	Any deep fry veg(0.5 oz)
Bamboo shoots	Beets	Any veg w/butter, marg
Broccoli	Brussels sprouts	Any veg w/cheese sauce
Butterbur	Carrots	Arrowhead
Cauliflower	Hubbard/winter squash	Baked beans
Crookneck/scallop squash	Hyacinth beans	Broad beans
Eggplant	Kale	Corn/creamed corn
Rhubarb	Leeks	Green peas/cowpeas
Sauerkraut	Mixed vegetables	Kidney/pinto beans
Spaghetti/summer squash	Navy beans	Lima beans
Spinach	Okra	Parsnips
String beans	Onions	Pigeon peas
Fresh or stewed tomatoes	Rutabagas	Soybeans
Turnips	Shellie beans	Succotash
Zucchini	Winged beans	Sweet potatoes/yams

(4.0 ounces)	(1.5 ounces)	(0.5 ounce)
Fresh fruit	Frozen yogurt (2.5 oz)	Cake and pastry
Gelatin dessert	Fudgsicles	Candy and chocolate
Gelatin w/fruit	Ice milk	Cookies
Lo cal gelatin (unlimited)	Popsicles (2.5 ounces)	Ice cream/sundae (1.0 oz)
Lo cal popsicle (unlimit)	Pudding	Pie (1.0 ounce)
Lo cal pudding	Sherbert	

DAILY MENU PLAN #3 -- 1400 CALORIES

BREAKFAST -- Choose 1 item from each section (i.e., choose 1 breakfast meat, 1 egg dish, and 1 juice). Select mostly "Light" foods.

Calorie Light	Calorie Moderate	Calorie Dense
(3.5 ounces)	(2.5 ounces)	(1.5 ounce)
Canadian bacon	Headcheese	Bacon (1.0 ounce)
Corned/roast beef hash	Regular ham	Blood sausage
Honey roll sausage, beef	Scrapple	Brown & serve sausage
Lean ham		Ham patties
New Eng. brand sausage		Other pork/beef sausage
Souse		Sirloin steak
(11.5 ounces)	(3.5 ounces)	(2.5 ounces)
Egg beaters	Fried eggs	Deviled eggs
Egg beater/cheese(4.5 oz)	Hard-boiled eggs	Egg yolks (1.5 ounces)
Egg whites	Omelets (3.0 ounces)	Quiche
	Other eggs	
	Poached eggs	
	Scrambled eggs	
	Soft-boiled eggs	
(4.5 ounces)	(3.5 ounces)	(1.5 ounce)
Apple cider	Apricot nectar	Coconut milk
Apple juice	Cranberry juice	
Blackberry juice	Cran-apple juice	
Grapefruit juice	Cran-apricot juice	
Grapefruit juice, sweetnd	Cran-grape juice	
Orange juice	Grape juice	
Orange-grapefruit juice	Orange-apricot juice	
Tangerine juice	Papaya nectar	
Tangelo juice	Passion fruit juice	
Tomato juice (9.5 ounces)	Peach or pear nectar	
	Pineapple juice	
	Pineapple-grapefrt juice	
	Pineapple-orange juice	
	Pine-orange-banana juice	
	Prune juice	

LUNCH -- Choose 1 item from each section. Select mostly "Light" foods.

Calorie Light	Calorie Moderate	Calorie Dense
(7.5 ounces)	(5.5 ounces)	(3.5 ounces)
Any 91% fat-free meat	Any 82% fat-free meat	All other lunch meat
Crab	Beef flank steak	All other pork
Fish canned in water	*Calf heart	Anything w/butter sauce
Lean ham	Lean lamb	Anything w/cream sauce
Lobster	*Liver	Anything with cheese
Other fish, not fried	Pork feet	Beef ribs
*Other organ meat	*Pork pancreas	Beef/pork tongue
Other seafood	Poultry, dark meat	Fried chicken/fried meat
Pork tenderloin, lean	Poultry with skin	Fried fish/fried seafood
Poultry, white w/gravy	Regular ham	Hamburger/meatloaf
Poultry, white w/o skin	Veal	Hot dog/sausage/kielbasa
Raw/steamed clams	Wild game	Other pork
Shrimp		Other steak/other beef
		Pork tail
*very high in cholesterol	*very high cholesterol	Poultry, dark w/skin

(6.5 ounces)	(4.0 ounces)	(3.0 ounces)
Bouillon (unlimited amt)	Soup, black bean	Soup, any chunky kind
Soup, beef mushroom	Soup, chicken dumpling	Soup, any made w/milk
Soup, beef noodle	Soup, cream of, w/water	Soup, bean w/bacon
Soup, chicken gumbo	Soup, pepper pot	Soup, bean w/franks
Soup, chicken noodle	Soup, tomato bisque	Soup, cheese
Soup, chicken vegetable	Soup, tomato with rice	Soup, chicken mushrm
Soup, chicken with rice		Soup, chili beef
Soup, Manh clam chowdr		Soup, N.E. clam chowdr
Soup, minestrone		Soup, pea green
Soup, mushrm w/barley		Soup, split pea w/ham
Soup, onion		Soup, tomato beef noodl
Soup, oyster stew w/watr		
Soup, Scotch broth		
Soup, tomato (w/water)		
Soup, turkey noodle		
Soup, turkey vegetable		
Soup, vegetable beef		
Soup, vegetarian vegetabl		

(4.5 ounces)	(2.5 ounces)	(1.5 ounce)
Fruit canned in juice	Bananas	Candied fruit
Fruit canned light syrup	Breadfruit	Coconut
Other fresh fruit	Crabapples	Dates
	Elderberries	Dried Fruit
	Fresh figs	Prunes
	Fruit canned hvy syrup	Raisins
	Passion fruit	
	Plantain	
	Sweetened fruit	

(10.5 ounces)	(6.0 ounces)	(3.5 ounces)
Cultured buttermilk	Chocolate milk	Eggnog
Low-fat milk	Coffee flavor milk	Hot cocoa made w/milk
Skim milk	Low-fat chocolate milk	Milk shake
	Whole goat milk	Whole sheep milk
	Whole milk	

DINNER -- Choose 1 item from each section. Select mostly "Light" foods.

Calorie Light	Calorie Moderate	Calorie Dense
(9.5 ounces)	(4.5 ounces)	(2.0 ounce)
Garden salad, no dressing	Salad with croutons	Any salad w/dressing
Salad with no-fat dressing	Salad with olives	Any salad w/mayonnaise
		Any salad with oil
		Chef salad/Caesar salad
(6.0 ounces)	(3.5 ounces)	(2.5 ounces)
Beef stew	Burritos	Cheese fondue
Casserole in tomato sauce	Chicken a la king	Chili con queso
Chili	Corned beef hash	Meatloaf
Diet entrees, except fried	Curry dishes with rice	Nachos
Pasta in tomato sauce	Enchiladas	Pasta in cream sauce
Shrimp creole	Macaroni and cheese	Pasta w/carbonara sauce
	Newburg dishes w/pasta	Stuffed potato skins
	Newburg dishes w/rice	Quiche
	Other casseroles	
	Other frozen entrees	
	Other pasta w/cheese	
	Other pasta w/meat	
	Pizza	
	Pot pies	
	Tacos	
	Tuna casserole	
(3.5 ounces)	(2.5 ounces)	(1.5 ounce)
Any rice/potato w/gravy	Any rice/potato w/butter	Any fried potatoes
Plain baked potato	Any rice/potato w/chees	Potato skins, baked/fried
Plain boiled potato	Baked potato, sour crm	
Plain brown rice	Beef flavored rice	
Plain white rice	Chicken flavored rice	
Scalloped potatoes	Chinese fried rice	
Spanish rice	Other flavored rice	

(9.5 ounces)	(4.5 ounces)	(2.5 ounces)
Asparagus	Acorn/butternut squash	Any deep fry veg(0.5 oz)
Bamboo shoots	Beets	Any veg w/butter, marg
Broccoli	Brussels sprouts	Any veg w/cheese sauce
Butterbur	Carrots	Arrowhead
Cauliflower	Hubbard/winter squash	Baked beans
Crookneck/scallop squash	Hyacinth beans	Broad beans
Eggplant	Kale	Corn/creamed corn
Rhubarb	Leeks	Green peas/cowpeas
Sauerkraut	Mixed vegetables	Kidney/pinto beans
Spaghetti/summer squash	Navy beans	Lima beans
Spinach	Okra	Parsnips
String beans	Onions	Pigeon peas
Fresh or stewed tomatoes	Rutabagas	Soybeans
Turnips	Shellie beans	Succotash
Zucchini	Winged beans	Sweet potatoes/yams

(4.5 ounces)	(1.5 ounce)	(0.5 ounce)
Fresh fruit	Frozen yogurt (3.0 oz)	Cake and pastry
Gelatin dessert	Fudgsicles	Candy and chocolate
Gelatin w/fruit	Ice milk	Cookies
Lo cal gelatin (unlimited)	Popsicles (3.0 ounces)	Ice cream/sundae (1.5 oz)
Lo cal popsicle (unlimit)	Pudding	Pie (1.5 ounce)
Lo cal pudding	Sherbert	

DAILY MENU PLAN #4 -- 1400 Calories

BREAKFAST -- Choose 1 item from each section (i.e., choose 1 breakfast bread product, 1 cereal, and 1 fruit). Select mostly "Light" foods.

Calorie Light	Calorie Moderate	Calorie Dense
(2.5 ounces)	(2.0 ounces)	(1.5 ounce)
French toast with syrup	Bagel with cream cheese	Biscuits with butter
Pancakes with syrup	Brown & serve rolls	Croissant
Plain bagel, any type	Coffee cake	Croissant with butter
Plain cornbread, homemd	English muffin w/butter	Danish pastry
Plain English muffins	Muffins, any type	Donuts, any type
Plain toast, low calorie	Pancakes w/butter,syrup	Matzo with butter
Toast w/low cal spread	Plain biscuits	
Waffles with syrup	Sweet rolls	
	Toast w/butter and jelly	
	Waffles w/butter, syrup	
(9.0 ounces)	(1.5 ounces)	(1.0 ounce)
Cream of wheat, cooked	*Bran cereals	*Granola-type cereals
Grits, cooked	*Flakes w/dried fruit	*Sugar-coated cereals
Malt-o-meal, cooked	*Other cereals	*High-sugar cereals
Maypo, cooked	*Plain flakes, any type	
Oatmeal, any type,cooked	*Wheat squares w/fruit	
Other hot cereal, cooked		
Ralston, cooked		
Wheatena, cooked	*Plus skim milk (4.5 oz)	*Plus skim milk (4.5 oz)
(3.5 ounces)	(2.5 ounces)	(0.5 ounce)
Fruit canned in juice	Bananas	Candied fruit
Fruit canned in lt syrup	Breadfruit	Coconut
Other fresh fruit	Crabapples	Dates
	Elderberries	Dried fruit
	Fresh figs	Prunes
	Fruit canned hvy syrup	Raisins
	Passion fruit	
	Plantain	
	Sweetened fruit	

LUNCH -- Choose 1 item from each section. Select mostly "Light" foods.

Calorie Light	Calorie Moderate	Calorie Dense
(6.0 ounces)	(4.5 ounces)	(4.0 ounces)
Sndwch,91% fat-free meat	Sndwch, 82-92% fat-free	Any croissant sandwich
Sandwich, grilled fish	Sandwich, regular ham	Any fried sandwich
Sandwich, grilled chicken		Any sandwich w/bacon
Sandwich, tuna (in water)		Any sandwich w/cheese
Sandwich, turkey		Any sandwich w/mayo
Sandwich, turkey breast		Burger/hot dog, all types
Sndwch, vegetarian(9.5oz)		Sandwich, meatball
		Sandwich, other meat
		Sndwch, p.b. &/or jelly
		Sandwich, submarine
(9.5 ounces)	(4.5 ounces)	(2.0 ounce)
Garden salad, no dressing	Salad with croutons	Any salad w/dressing
Salad with no-fat dressing	Salad with olives	Any salad w/mayonnaise
		Any salad with oil
		Chef salad/Caesar salad
(6.0 ounces)	(4.0 ounces)	(1.0 ounce)
Apple cider	Apricot nectar	Coconut milk
Apple juice	Cranberry juice	
Blackberry juice	Cran-apple juice	
Grapefruit juice	Cran-apricot juice	
Grapefruit juice, sweetnd	Cran-grape juice	
Orange juice	Grape juice	
Orange-grapefruit juice	Orange-apricot juice	
Tangerine juice	Papaya nectar	
Tangelo juice	Passion fruit juice	
Tomato juice (10.0 oz)	Peach nectar	
	Pear nectar	
	Pineapple juice	
	Pineapple-grapefrt juice	
	Pineapple-orange juice	
	Pine-orange-banana juice	
	Prune juice	

(5.5 ounces)	(2.0 ounces)	(1.5 ounces)
Cottage cheese, any type	Feta cheese	All other cheese
Lite ricotta	Neufchatel cheese	
Frozen yogurt	Part-skim mozzarella	
Yogurt, any type	Ricotta cheese	
	Skim mozzarella cheese	

DINNER -- Choose 1 item from each section. Select mostly "Light" foods.

Calorie Light	Calorie Moderate	Calorie Dense
(9.5 ounces)	(4.5 ounces)	(2.0 ounce)
Garden salad, no dressing	Salad with croutons	Any salad w/dressing
Salad with no-fat dressing	Salad with olives	Any salad w/mayonnaise
		Any salad with oil
		Chef salad/Caesar salad
(4.5 ounces)	(3.5 ounces)	(2.5 ounces)
Any 91% fat-free meat	Any 82% fat-free meat	All other lunch meat
Crab	Beef flank steak	All other pork
Fish canned in water	*Calf heart	Anything w/butter sauce
Lean ham	Lean lamb	Anything w/cream sauce
Lobster	*Liver	Anything with cheese
Other fish, not fried	Pork feet	Beef ribs
*Other organ meat	*Pork pancreas	Beef/pork tongue
Other seafood	Poultry, dark meat	Fried chicken/fried meat
Pork tenderloin, lean	Poultry with skin	Fried fish/fried seafood
Poultry, white w/gravy	Regular ham	Hamburger/meatloaf
Poultry, white w/o skin	Veal	Hot dog/sausage/kielbasa
Raw/steamed clams	Wild game	Other pork
Shrimp		Other steak/other beef
		Pork tail
*very high in cholesterol	*very high cholesterol	Poultry, dark w/skin
(1.5 ounces)	(1.5 ounce)	(0.5 ounce)
Plain bagels, any type	Bagels w/cream cheese	All other crackers
Cornbread	Bread/rolls with butter	All other nuts
Plain muffins, any type	Croissants	Cheetos/cheese curls
Plain bread/rolls	Honey-coated grahams	Chex snack mix
Roasted chestnuts	Matzo/bread sticks	Chips, any variety
	Oyster crackers	Microwave popcorn
	Plain air-pop popcorn	Popcorn, oil popped
	Plain graham crackers	Popcorn with butter
	Pretzels	Seeds, any type
	Soda crackers	
	Triscuit crackers	

(9.5 ounces)	(4.5 ounces)	(2.5 ounces)
Asparagus	Acorn/butternut squash	Any deep fry veg(0.5 oz)
Bamboo shoots	Beets	Any veg w/butter, marg
Broccoli	Brussels sprouts	Any veg w/cheese sauce
Butterbur	Carrots	Arrowhead
Cauliflower	Hubbard/winter squash	Baked beans
Crookneck/scallop squash	Hyacinth beans	Broad beans
Eggplant	Kale	Corn/creamed corn
Rhubarb	Leeks	Green peas/cowpeas
Sauerkraut	Mixed vegetables	Kidney/pinto beans
Spaghetti/summer squash	Navy beans	Lima beans
Spinach	Okra	Parsnips
String beans	Onions	Pigeon peas
Fresh or stewed tomatoes	Rutabagas	Soybeans
Turnips	Shellie beans	Succotash
Zucchini	Winged beans	Sweet potatoes/yams

(4.5 ounces)	(1.5 ounces)	(0.5 ounce)
Fresh fruit	Frozen yogurt (3.0 oz)	Cake and pastry
Gelatin dessert	Fudgsicles	Candy and chocolate
Gelatin w/fruit	Ice milk	Cookies
Lo cal gelatin (unlimited)	Popsicles (3.0 ounces)	Ice cream/sundae (1.5 oz)
Lo cal popsicle (unlimit)	Pudding	Pie (1.5 ounce)
Lo cal pudding	Sherbert	

DAILY MENU PLAN #5 -- 1600 CALORIES

BREAKFAST -- Choose 1 item from each section (i.e., choose 1 breakfast meat, 1 egg dish, and 1 juice). Select mostly "Light" foods.

Calorie Light	Calorie Moderate	Calorie Dense
(3.5 ounces)	(3.0 ounces)	(1.5 ounce)
Canadian bacon	Headcheese	Bacon (1.5 ounces)
Corned/roast beef hash	Regular ham	Blood sausage
Honey roll sausage, beef	Scrapple	Brown & serve sausage
Lean ham		Ham patties
New Eng. brand sausage		Other pork/beef sausage
Souse		Sirloin steak
(13.5 ounces)	(4.0 ounces)	(2.5 ounces)
Egg beaters	Fried eggs	Deviled eggs
Egg beater/cheese(5.5 oz)	Hard-boiled eggs	Egg yolks (1.5 ounces)
Egg whites	Omelets (3.5 ounces)	Quiche
	Other eggs	
	Poached eggs	
	Scrambled eggs	
	Soft-boiled eggs	
(5.5 ounces)	(4.0 ounces)	(1.0 ounce)
Apple cider	Apricot nectar	Coconut milk
Apple juice	Cranberry juice	
Blackberry juice	Cran-apple juice	
Grapefruit juice	Cran-apricot juice	
Grapefruit juice, sweetnd	Cran-grape juice	
Orange juice	Grape juice	
Orange-grapefruit juice	Orange-apricot juice	
Tangerine juice	Papaya nectar	
Tangelo juice	Passion fruit juice	
Tomato juice (10.5 oz)	Peach or pear nectar	
	Pineapple juice	
	Pineapple-grapefrt juice	
	Pineapple-orange juice	
	Pine-orange-banana juice	
	Prune juice	

LUNCH -- Choose 1 item from each section. Select mostly "Light" foods.

Calorie Light	Calorie Moderate	Calorie Dense
(8.5 ounces)	(6.5 ounces)	(4.5 ounces)
Any 91% fat-free meat	Any 82% fat-free meat	All other lunch meat
Crab	Beef flank steak	All other pork
Fish canned in water	*Calf heart	Anything w/butter sauce
Lean ham	Lean lamb	Anything w/cream sauce
Lobster	*Liver	Anything with cheese
Other fish, not fried	Pork feet	Beef ribs
*Other organ meat	*Pork pancreas	Beef/pork tongue
Other seafood	Poultry, dark meat	Fried chicken/fried meat
Pork tenderloin, lean	Poultry with skin	Fried fish/fried seafood
Poultry, white w/gravy	Regular ham	Hamburger/meatloaf
Poultry, white w/o skin	Veal	Hot dog/sausage/kielbasa
Raw/steamed clams	Wild game	Other pork
Shrimp		Other steak/other beef
		Pork tail
*very high in cholesterol	*very high cholesterol	Poultry, dark w/skin
(7.5 ounces)	(4.5 ounces)	(3.5 ounces)
Bouillon (unlimited amt)	Soup, black bean	Soup, any chunky kind
Soup, beef mushroom	Soup, chicken dumpling	Soup, any made w/milk
Soup, beef noodle	Soup, cream of, w/water	Soup, bean w/bacon
Soup, chicken gumbo	Soup, pepper pot	Soup, bean w/franks
Soup, chicken noodle	Soup, tomato bisque	Soup, cheese
Soup, chicken vegetable	Soup, tomato with rice	Soup, chicken mushrm
Soup, chicken with rice		Soup, chili beef
Soup, Manh clam chowdr		Soup, N.E. clam chowdr
Soup, minestrone		Soup, pea green
Soup, mushrm w/barley		Soup, split pea w/ham
Soup, onion		Soup, tomato beef noodl
Soup, oyster stew w/watr		
Soup, Scotch broth		
Soup, tomato (w/water)		
Soup, turkey noodle		
Soup, turkey vegetable		
Soup, vegetable beef		
Soup, vegetarian vegetabl		

(5.5 ounces)	(3.5 ounces)	(1.0 ounce)
Fruit canned in juice	Bananas	Candied fruit
Fruit canned light syrup	Breadfruit	Coconut
Other fresh fruit	Crabapples	Dates
	Elderberries	Dried Fruit
	Fresh figs	Prunes
	Fruit canned hvy syrup	Raisins
	Passion fruit	
	Plantain	
	Sweetened fruit	

(12.0 ounces)	(6.5 ounces)	(4.0 ounces)
Cultured buttermilk	Chocolate milk	Eggnog
Low-fat milk	Coffee flavor milk	Hot cocoa made w/milk
Skim milk	Low-fat chocolate milk	Milk shake
	Whole goat milk	Whole sheep milk
	Whole milk	

DINNER -- Choose 1 item from each section. Select mostly "Light" foods.

Calorie Light	Calorie Moderate	Calorie Dense
(10.5 ounces)	(5.0 ounces)	(2.5 ounce)
Garden salad, no dressing	Salad with croutons	Any salad w/dressing
Salad with no-fat dressing	Salad with olives	Any salad w/mayonnaise
		Any salad with oil
		Chef salad/Caesar salad
(6.5 ounces)	(4.0 ounces)	(2.5 ounces)
Beef stew	Burritos	Cheese fondue
Casserole in tomato sauce	Chicken a la king	Chili con queso
Chili	Corned beef hash	Meatloaf
Diet entrees, except fried	Curry dishes with rice	Nachos
Pasta in tomato sauce	Enchiladas	Pasta in cream sauce
Shrimp creole	Macaroni and cheese	Pasta w/carbonara sauce
	Newburg dishes w/pasta	Stuffed potato skins
	Newburg dishes w/rice	Quiche
	Other casseroles	
	Other frozen entrees	
	Other pasta w/cheese	
	Other pasta w/meat	
	Pizza	
	Pot pies	
	Tacos	
	Tuna casserole	
(4.0 ounces)	(2.5 ounces)	(1.5 ounces)
Any rice/potato w/gravy	Any rice/potato w/butter	Any fried potatoes
Plain baked potato	Any rice/potato w/chees	Potato skins, baked/fried
Plain boiled potato	Baked potato, sour crm	
Plain brown rice	Beef flavored rice	
Plain white rice	Chicken flavored rice	
Scalloped potatoes	Chinese fried rice	
Spanish rice	Other flavored rice	

(10.5 ounces)	(5.5 ounces)	(2.5 ounces)
Asparagus	Acorn/butternut squash	Any deep fry veg(0.5 oz)
Bamboo shoots	Beets	Any veg w/butter, marg
Broccoli	Brussels sprouts	Any veg w/cheese sauce
Butterbur	Carrots	Arrowhead
Cauliflower	Hubbard/winter squash	Baked beans
Crookneck/scallop squash	Hyacinth beans	Broad beans
Eggplant	Kale	Corn/creamed corn
Rhubarb	Leeks	Green peas/cowpeas
Sauerkraut	Mixed vegetables	Kidney/pinto beans
Spaghetti/summer squash	Navy beans	Lima beans
Spinach	Okra	Parsnips
String beans	Onions	Pigeon peas
Fresh or stewed tomatoes	Rutabagas	Soybeans
Turnips	Shellie beans	Succotash
Zucchini	Winged beans	Sweet potatoes/yams

(5.5 ounces)	(2.0 ounce)	(0.5 ounce)
Fresh fruit	Frozen yogurt (3.5 oz)	Cake and pastry
Gelatin dessert	Fudgsicles	Candy and chocolate
Gelatin w/fruit	Ice milk	Cookies
Lo cal gelatin (unlimited)	Popsicles (3.5 ounces)	Ice cream/sundae (1.5 oz)
Lo cal popsicle (unlimit)	Pudding	Pie (1.5 ounces)
Lo cal pudding	Sherbert	

DAILY MENU PLAN #6 -- 1600 Calories

BREAKFAST -- Choose 1 item from each section (i.e., choose 1 breakfast bread product, 1 cereal, and 1 fruit). Select mostly "Light" foods.

Calorie Light	Calorie Moderate	Calorie Dense
(3.0 ounces)	(2.0 ounces)	(1.5 ounce)
French toast with syrup	Bagel with cream cheese	Biscuits with butter
Pancakes with syrup	Brown & serve rolls	Croissant
Plain bagel, any type	Coffee cake	Croissant with butter
Plain cornbread, homemd	English muffin w/butter	Danish pastry
Plain English muffins	Muffins, any type	Donuts, any type
Plain toast, low calorie	Pancakes w/butter,syrup	Matzo with butter
Toast w/low cal spread	Plain biscuits	
Waffles with syrup	Sweet rolls	
	Toast w/butter and jelly	
	Waffles w/butter, syrup	
(10.5 ounces)	(1.5 ounces)	(1.0 ounce)
Cream of wheat, cooked	*Bran cereals	*Granola-type cereals
Grits, cooked	*Flakes w/dried fruit	*Sugar-coated cereals
Malt-o-meal, cooked	*Other cereals	*High-sugar cereals
Maypo, cooked	*Plain flakes, any type	
Oatmeal, any type,cooked	*Wheat squares w/fruit	
Other hot cereal, cooked		
Ralston, cooked		
Wheatena, cooked	*Plus skim milk (5.5 oz)	*Plus skim milk (5.5 oz)
(4.5 ounces)	(2.5 ounces)	(1.5 ounce)
Fruit canned in juice	Bananas	Candied fruit
Fruit canned in lt syrup	Breadfruit	Coconut
Other fresh fruit	Crabapples	Dates
	Elderberries	Dried fruit
	Fresh figs	Prunes
	Fruit canned hvy syrup	Raisins
	Passion fruit	
	Plantain	
	Sweetened fruit	

LUNCH -- Choose 1 item from each section. Select mostly "Light" foods.

Calorie Light	Calorie Moderate	Calorie Dense
(6.5 ounces)	(5.5 ounces)	(4.5 ounces)
Sndwch,91% fat-free meat	Sndwch, 82-92% fat-free	Any croissant sandwich
Sandwich, grilled fish	Sandwich, regular ham	Any fried sandwich
Sandwich, grilled chicken		Any sandwich w/bacon
Sandwich, tuna (in water)		Any sandwich w/cheese
Sandwich, turkey		Any sandwich w/mayo
Sandwich, turkey breast		Burger/hot dog, all types
Sndwch, vegetarn(10.5oz)		Sandwich, meatball
		Sandwich, other meat
		Sndwch, p.b. &/or jelly
		Sandwich, submarine
(10.5 ounces)	(5.0 ounces)	(2.5 ounce)
Garden salad, no dressing	Salad with croutons	Any salad w/dressing
Salad with no-fat dressing	Salad with olives	Any salad w/mayonnaise
		Any salad with oil
		Chef salad/Caesar salad
(6.5 ounces)	(4.5 ounces)	(1.5 ounce)
Apple cider	Apricot nectar	Coconut milk
Apple juice	Cranberry juice	
Blackberry juice	Cran-apple juice	
Grapefruit juice	Cran-apricot juice	
Grapefruit juice, sweetnd	Cran-grape juice	
Orange juice	Grape juice	
Orange-grapefruit juice	Orange-apricot juice	
Tangerine juice	Papaya nectar	
Tangelo juice	Passion fruit juice	
Tomato juice (13.0 oz)	Peach nectar	
	Pear nectar	
	Pineapple juice	
	Pineapple-grapefrt juice	
	Pineapple-orange juice	
	Pine-orange-banana juice	
	Prune juice	

(6.0 ounces)	(2.5 ounces)	(1.5 ounces)
Cottage cheese, any type	Feta cheese	All other cheese
Lite ricotta	Neufchatel cheese	
Frozen yogurt	Part-skim mozzarella	
Yogurt, any type	Ricotta cheese	
	Skim mozzarella cheese	

DINNER -- Choose 1 item from each section. Select mostly "Light" foods.

Calorie Light	Calorie Moderate	Calorie Dense
(10.5 ounces)	(5.0 ounces)	(2.5 ounces)
Garden salad, no dressing	Salad with croutons	Any salad w/dressing
Salad with no-fat dressing	Salad with olives	Any salad w/mayonnaise
		Any salad with oil
		Chef salad/Caesar salad
(5.5 ounces)	(4.0 ounces)	(2.5 ounces)
Any 91% fat-free meat	Any 82% fat-free meat	All other lunch meat
Crab	Beef flank steak	All other pork
Fish canned in water	*Calf heart	Anything w/butter sauce
Lean ham	Lean lamb	Anything w/cream sauce
Lobster	*Liver	Anything with cheese
Other fish, not fried	Pork feet	Beef ribs
*Other organ meat	*Pork pancreas	Beef/pork tongue
Other seafood	Poultry, dark meat	Fried chicken/fried meat
Pork tenderloin, lean	Poultry with skin	Fried fish/fried seafood
Poultry, white w/gravy	Regular ham	Hamburger/meatloaf
Poultry, white w/o skin	Veal	Hot dog/sausage/kielbasa
Raw/steamed clams	Wild game	Other pork
Shrimp		Other steak/other beef
		Pork tail
*very high in cholesterol	*very high cholesterol	Poultry, dark w/skin
(1.5 ounces)	(1.0 ounce)	(0.5 ounce)
Plain bagels, any type	Bagels w/cream cheese	All other crackers
Cornbread	Bread/rolls with butter	All other nuts
Plain muffins, any type	Croissants	Cheetos/cheese curls
Plain bread/rolls	Honey-coated grahams	Chex snack mix
Roasted chestnuts	Matzo/bread sticks	Chips, any variety
	Oyster crackers	Microwave popcorn
	Plain air-pop popcorn	Popcorn, oil popped
	Plain graham crackers	Popcorn with butter
	Pretzels	Seeds, any type
	Soda crackers	
	Triscuit crackers	

(10.5 ounces)	(5.5 ounces)	(2.5 ounces)
Asparagus	Acorn/butternut squash	Any deep fry veg(0.5 oz)
Bamboo shoots	Beets	Any veg w/butter, marg
Broccoli	Brussels sprouts	Any veg w/cheese sauce
Butterbur	Carrots	Arrowhead
Cauliflower	Hubbard/winter squash	Baked beans
Crookneck/scallop squash	Hyacinth beans	Broad beans
Eggplant	Kale	Corn/creamed corn
Rhubarb	Leeks	Green peas/cowpeas
Sauerkraut	Mixed vegetables	Kidney/pinto beans
Spaghetti/summer squash	Navy beans	Lima beans
Spinach	Okra	Parsnips
String beans	Onions	Pigeon peas
Fresh or stewed tomatoes	Rutabagas	Soybeans
Turnips	Shellie beans	Succotash
Zucchini	Winged beans	Sweet potatoes/yams

(5.5 ounces)	(2.0 ounces)	(0.5 ounce)
Fresh fruit	Frozen yogurt (3.5 oz)	Cake and pastry
Gelatin dessert	Fudgsicles	Candy and chocolate
Gelatin w/fruit	Ice milk	Cookies
Lo cal gelatin (unlimited)	Popsicles (3.5 ounces)	Ice cream/sundae (1.5 oz)
Lo cal popsicle (unlimit)	Pudding	Pie (1.5 ounces)
Lo cal pudding	Sherbert	

DAILY MENU PLAN #7 -- 1800 CALORIES

BREAKFAST -- Choose 1 item from each section (i.e., choose 1 breakfast meat, 1 egg dish, and 1 juice). Select mostly "Light" foods.

Calorie Light	Calorie Moderate	Calorie Dense
(4.0 ounces)	(3.5 ounces)	(2.0 ounce)
Canadian bacon	Headcheese	Bacon (1.5 ounces)
Corned/roast beef hash	Regular ham	Blood sausage
Honey roll sausage, beef	Scrapple	Brown & serve sausage
Lean ham		Ham patties
New Eng. brand sausage		Other pork/beef sausage
Souse		Sirloin steak
(15.0 ounces)	(4.5 ounces)	(3.0 ounces)
Egg beaters	Fried eggs	Deviled eggs
Egg beater/cheese(6.0 oz)	Hard-boiled eggs	Egg yolks (2.0 ounces)
Egg whites	Omelets (3.5 ounces)	Quiche
	Other eggs	
	Poached eggs	
	Scrambled eggs	
	Soft-boiled eggs	
(6.0 ounces)	(4.5 ounces)	(1.0 ounce)
Apple cider	Apricot nectar	Coconut milk
Apple juice	Cranberry juice	
Blackberry juice	Cran-apple juice	
Grapefruit juice	Cran-apricot juice	
Grapefruit juice, sweetnd	Cran-grape juice	
Orange juice	Grape juice	
Orange-grapefruit juice	Orange-apricot juice	
Tangerine juice	Papaya nectar	
Tangelo juice	Passion fruit juice	
Tomato juice (12.0 oz)	Peach or pear nectar	
	Pineapple juice	
	Pineapple-grapefrt juice	
	Pineapple-orange juice	
	Pine-orange-banana juice	
	Prune juice	

LUNCH -- Choose 1 item from each section. Select mostly "Light" foods.

Calorie Light	Calorie Moderate	Calorie Dense
(10.0 ounces)	(7.5 ounces)	(5.0 ounces)
Any 91% fat-free meat	Any 82% fat-free meat	All other lunch meat
Crab	Beef flank steak	All other pork
Fish canned in water	*Calf heart	Anything w/butter sauce
Lean ham	Lean lamb	Anything w/cream sauce
Lobster	*Liver	Anything with cheese
Other fish, not fried	Pork feet	Beef ribs
*Other organ meat	*Pork pancreas	Beef/pork tongue
Other seafood	Poultry, dark meat	Fried chicken/fried meat
Pork tenderloin, lean	Poultry with skin	Fried fish/fried seafood
Poultry, white w/gravy	Regular ham	Hamburger/meatloaf
Poultry, white w/o skin	Veal	Hot dog/sausage/kielbasa
Raw/steamed clams	Wild game	Other pork
Shrimp		Other steak/other beef
		Pork tail
*very high in cholesterol	*very high cholesterol	Poultry, dark w/skin

Calorie Light	Calorie Moderate	Calorie Dense
(8.5 ounces)	(5.5 ounces)	(3.5 ounces)
Bouillon (unlimited amt)	Soup, black bean	Soup, any chunky kind
Soup, beef mushroom	Soup, chicken dumpling	Soup, any made w/milk
Soup, beef noodle	Soup, cream of, w/water	Soup, bean w/bacon
Soup, chicken gumbo	Soup, pepper pot	Soup, bean w/franks
Soup, chicken noodle	Soup, tomato bisque	Soup, cheese
Soup, chicken vegetable	Soup, tomato with rice	Soup, chicken mushrm
Soup, chicken with rice		Soup, chili beef
Soup, Manh clam chowdr		Soup, N.E. clam chowdr
Soup, minestrone		Soup, pea green
Soup, mushrm w/barley		Soup, split pea w/ham
Soup, onion		Soup, tomato beef noodl
Soup, oyster stew w/watr		
Soup, Scotch broth		
Soup, tomato (w/water)		
Soup, turkey noodle		
Soup, turkey vegetable		
Soup, vegetable beef		
Soup, vegetarian vegetabl		

(6.0 ounces)	(4.0 ounces)	(1.0 ounce)
Fruit canned in juice	Bananas	Candied fruit
Fruit canned light syrup	Breadfruit	Coconut
Other fresh fruit	Crabapples	Dates
	Elderberries	Dried Fruit
	Fresh figs	Prunes
	Fruit canned hvy syrup	Raisins
	Passion fruit	
	Plantain	
	Sweetened fruit	

(13.5 ounces)	(7.5 ounces)	(4.5 ounces)
Cultured buttermilk	Chocolate milk	Eggnog
Low-fat milk	Coffee flavor milk	Hot cocoa made w/milk
Skim milk	Low-fat chocolate milk	Milk shake
	Whole goat milk	Whole sheep milk
	Whole milk	

DINNER -- Choose 1 item from each section. Select mostly "Light" foods.

Calorie Light	Calorie Moderate	Calorie Dense
(12.0 ounces)	(5.5 ounces)	(2.5 ounce)
Garden salad, no dressing	Salad with croutons	Any salad w/dressing
Salad with no-fat dressing	Salad with olives	Any salad w/mayonnaise
		Any salad with oil
		Chef salad/Caesar salad
(7.5 ounces)	(4.5 ounces)	(3.0 ounces)
Beef stew	Burritos	Cheese fondue
Casserole in tomato sauce	Chicken a la king	Chili con queso
Chili	Corned beef hash	Meatloaf
Diet entrees, except fried	Curry dishes with rice	Nachos
Pasta in tomato sauce	Enchiladas	Pasta in cream sauce
Shrimp creole	Macaroni and cheese	Pasta w/carbonara sauce
	Newburg dishes w/pasta	Stuffed potato skins
	Newburg dishes w/rice	Quiche
	Other casseroles	
	Other frozen entrees	
	Other pasta w/cheese	
	Other pasta w/meat	
	Pizza	
	Pot pies	
	Tacos	
	Tuna casserole	
(4.5 ounces)	(3.0 ounces)	(1.5 ounces)
Any rice/potato w/gravy	Any rice/potato w/butter	Any fried potatoes
Plain baked potato	Any rice/potato w/chees	Potato skins, baked/fried
Plain boiled potato	Baked potato, sour crm	
Plain brown rice	Beef flavored rice	
Plain white rice	Chicken flavored rice	
Scalloped potatoes	Chinese fried rice	
Spanish rice	Other flavored rice	

(12.0 ounces)	(6.0 ounces)	(3.0 ounces)
Asparagus	Acorn/butternut squash	Any deep fry veg(1.5 oz)
Bamboo shoots	Beets	Any veg w/butter, marg
Broccoli	Brussels sprouts	Any veg w/cheese sauce
Butterbur	Carrots	Arrowhead
Cauliflower	Hubbard/winter squash	Baked beans
Crookneck/scallop squash	Hyacinth beans	Broad beans
Eggplant	Kale	Corn/creamed corn
Rhubarb	Leeks	Green peas/cowpeas
Sauerkraut	Mixed vegetables	Kidney/pinto beans
Spaghetti/summer squash	Navy beans	Lima beans
Spinach	Okra	Parsnips
String beans	Onions	Pigeon peas
Fresh or stewed tomatoes	Rutabagas	Soybeans
Turnips	Shellie beans	Succotash
Zucchini	Winged beans	Sweet potatoes/yams

(6.0 ounces)	(2.5 ounce)	(1.5 ounce)
Fresh fruit	Frozen yogurt (4.0 oz)	Cake and pastry
Gelatin dessert	Fudgsicles	Candy and chocolate
Gelatin w/fruit	Ice milk	Cookies
Lo cal gelatin (unlimited)	Popsicles (4.0 ounces)	Ice cream/sundae
Lo cal popsicle (unlimit)	Pudding	Pie
Lo cal pudding	Sherbert	

DAILY MENU PLAN #8 -- 1800 Calories

BREAKFAST -- Choose 1 item from each section (i.e., choose 1 breakfast bread product, 1 cereal, and 1 fruit). Select mostly "Light" foods.

Calorie Light	Calorie Moderate	Calorie Dense
(3.5 ounces)	(2.5 ounces)	(1.5 ounce)
French toast with syrup	Bagel with cream cheese	Biscuits with butter
Pancakes with syrup	Brown & serve rolls	Croissant
Plain bagel, any type	Coffee cake	Croissant with butter
Plain cornbread, homemd	English muffin w/butter	Danish pastry
Plain English muffins	Muffins, any type	Donuts, any type
Plain toast, low calorie	Pancakes w/butter,syrup	Matzo with butter
Toast w/low cal spread	Plain biscuits	
Waffles with syrup	Sweet rolls	
	Toast w/butter and jelly	
	Waffles w/butter, syrup	
(11.5 ounces)	(1.5 ounces)	(1.5 ounce)
Cream of wheat, cooked	*Bran cereals	*Granola-type cereals
Grits, cooked	*Flakes w/dried fruit	*Sugar-coated cereals
Malt-o-meal, cooked	*Other cereals	*High-sugar cereals
Maypo, cooked	*Plain flakes, any type	
Oatmeal, any type,cooked	*Wheat squares w/fruit	
Other hot cereal, cooked		
Ralston, cooked		
Wheatena, cooked	*Plus skim milk (6.0 oz)	*Plus skim milk (6.0 oz)
(5.0 ounces)	(3.0 ounces)	(1.0 ounce)
Fruit canned in juice	Bananas	Candied fruit
Fruit canned in lt syrup	Breadfruit	Coconut
Other fresh fruit	Crabapples	Dates
	Elderberries	Dried fruit
	Fresh figs	Prunes
	Fruit canned hvy syrup	Raisins
	Passion fruit	
	Plantain	
	Sweetened fruit	

LUNCH -- Choose 1 item from each section. Select mostly "Light" foods.

Calorie Light	Calorie Moderate	Calorie Dense
(7.5 ounces)	(6.0 ounces)	(5.5 ounces)
Sndwch,91% fat-free meat	Sndwch, 82-92% fat-free	Any croissant sandwich
Sandwich, grilled fish	Sandwich, regular ham	Any fried sandwich
Sandwich, grilled chicken		Any sandwich w/bacon
Sandwich, tuna (in water)		Any sandwich w/cheese
Sandwich, turkey		Any sandwich w/mayo
Sandwich, turkey breast		Burger/hot dog, all types
Sndwch, vegetarn(12.0oz)		Sandwich, meatball
		Sandwich, other meat
		Sndwch, p.b. &/or jelly
		Sandwich, submarine

Calorie Light	Calorie Moderate	Calorie Dense
(12.0 ounces)	(5.5 ounces)	(2.5 ounce)
Garden salad, no dressing	Salad with croutons	Any salad w/dressing
Salad with no-fat dressing	Salad with olives	Any salad w/mayonnaise
		Any salad with oil
		Chef salad/Caesar salad

Calorie Light	Calorie Moderate	Calorie Dense
(7.5 ounces)	(5.5 ounces)	(1.5 ounce)
Apple cider	Apricot nectar	Coconut milk
Apple juice	Cranberry juice	
Blackberry juice	Cran-apple juice	
Grapefruit juice	Cran-apricot juice	
Grapefruit juice, sweetnd	Cran-grape juice	
Orange juice	Grape juice	
Orange-grapefruit juice	Orange-apricot juice	
Tangerine juice	Papaya nectar	
Tangelo juice	Passion fruit juice	
Tomato juice (15.0 oz)	Peach nectar	
	Pear nectar	
	Pineapple juice	
	Pineapple-grapefrt juice	
	Pineapple-orange juice	
	Pine-orange-banana juice	
	Prune juice	

(7.0 ounces)	(2.5 ounces)	(1.5 ounces)
Cottage cheese, any type	Feta cheese	All other cheese
Lite ricotta	Neufchatel cheese	
Frozen yogurt	Part-skim mozzarella	
Yogurt, any type	Ricotta cheese	
	Skim mozzarella cheese	

DINNER -- Choose 1 item from each section. Select mostly "Light" foods.

Calorie Light	Calorie Moderate	Calorie Dense
(12.0 ounces)	(5.5 ounces)	(2.5 ounces)
Garden salad, no dressing	Salad with croutons	Any salad w/dressing
Salad with no-fat dressing	Salad with olives	Any salad w/mayonnaise
		Any salad with oil
		Chef salad/Caesar salad
(6.0 ounces)	(4.5 ounces)	(3.0 ounces)
Any 91% fat-free meat	Any 82% fat-free meat	All other lunch meat
Crab	Beef flank steak	All other pork
Fish canned in water	*Calf heart	Anything w/butter sauce
Lean ham	Lean lamb	Anything w/cream sauce
Lobster	*Liver	Anything with cheese
Other fish, not fried	Pork feet	Beef ribs
*Other organ meat	*Pork pancreas	Beef/pork tongue
Other seafood	Poultry, dark meat	Fried chicken/fried meat
Pork tenderloin, lean	Poultry with skin	Fried fish/fried seafood
Poultry, white w/gravy	Regular ham	Hamburger/meatloaf
Poultry, white w/o skin	Veal	Hot dog/sausage/kielbasa
Raw/steamed clams	Wild game	Other pork
Shrimp		Other steak/other beef
		Pork tail
*very high in cholesterol	*very high cholesterol	Poultry, dark w/skin
(1.5 ounces)	(1.0 ounce)	(0.5 ounce)
Plain bagels, any type	Bagels w/cream cheese	All other crackers
Cornbread	Bread/rolls with butter	All other nuts
Plain muffins, any type	Croissants	Cheetos/cheese curls
Plain bread/rolls	Honey-coated grahams	Chex snack mix
Roasted chestnuts	Matzo/bread sticks	Chips, any variety
	Oyster crackers	Microwave popcorn
	Plain air-pop popcorn	Popcorn, oil popped
	Plain graham crackers	Popcorn with butter
	Pretzels	Seeds, any type
	Soda crackers	
	Triscuit crackers	

(12.0 ounces)	(6.0 ounces)	(3.0 ounces)
Asparagus	Acorn/butternut squash	Any deep fry veg(1.5 oz)
Bamboo shoots	Beets	Any veg w/butter, marg
Broccoli	Brussels sprouts	Any veg w/cheese sauce
Butterbur	Carrots	Arrowhead
Cauliflower	Hubbard/winter squash	Baked beans
Crookneck/scallop squash	Hyacinth beans	Broad beans
Eggplant	Kale	Corn/creamed corn
Rhubarb	Leeks	Green peas/cowpeas
Sauerkraut	Mixed vegetables	Kidney/pinto beans
Spaghetti/summer squash	Navy beans	Lima beans
Spinach	Okra	Parsnips
String beans	Onions	Pigeon peas
Fresh or stewed tomatoes	Rutabagas	Soybeans
Turnips	Shellie beans	Succotash
Zucchini	Winged beans	Sweet potatoes/yams

(6.0 ounces)	(2.5 ounces)	(1.5 ounce)
Fresh fruit	Frozen yogurt (3.5 oz)	Cake and pastry
Gelatin dessert	Fudgsicles	Candy and chocolate
Gelatin w/fruit	Ice milk	Cookies
Lo cal gelatin (unlimited)	Popsicles (3.5 ounces)	Ice cream/sundae
Lo cal popsicle (unlimit)	Pudding	Pie
Lo cal pudding	Sherbert	

DAILY MENU PLAN #9 -- 2000 CALORIES

BREAKFAST -- Choose 1 item from each section (i.e., choose 1 breakfast meat, 1 egg dish, and 1 juice). Select mostly "Light" foods.

Calorie Light	Calorie Moderate	Calorie Dense
(4.5 ounces)	(3.5 ounces)	(2.5 ounce)
Canadian bacon	Headcheese	Bacon (1.5 ounces)
Corned/roast beef hash	Regular ham	Blood sausage
Honey roll sausage, beef	Scrapple	Brown & serve sausage
Lean ham		Ham patties
New Eng. brand sausage		Other pork/beef sausage
Souse		Sirloin steak
(16.5 ounces)	(5.0 ounces)	(3.5 ounces)
Egg beaters	Fried eggs	Deviled eggs
Egg beater/cheese(6.5 oz)	Hard-boiled eggs	Egg yolks (2.5 ounces)
Egg whites	Omelets (4.0 ounces)	Quiche
	Other eggs	
	Poached eggs	
	Scrambled eggs	
	Soft-boiled eggs	
(6.5 ounces)	(5.0 ounces)	(1.5 ounce)
Apple cider	Apricot nectar	Coconut milk
Apple juice	Cranberry juice	
Blackberry juice	Cran-apple juice	
Grapefruit juice	Cran-apricot juice	
Grapefruit juice, sweetnd	Cran-grape juice	
Orange juice	Grape juice	
Orange-grapefruit juice	Orange-apricot juice	
Tangerine juice	Papaya nectar	
Tangelo juice	Passion fruit juice	
Tomato juice (13.5 oz)	Peach or pear nectar	
	Pineapple juice	
	Pineapple-grapefrt juice	
	Pineapple-orange juice	
	Pine-orange-banana juice	
	Prune juice	

LUNCH -- Choose 1 item from each section. Select mostly "Light" foods.

Calorie Light	Calorie Moderate	Calorie Dense
(11.0 ounces)	(8.0 ounces)	(5.5 ounces)
Any 91% fat-free meat	Any 82% fat-free meat	All other lunch meat
Crab	Beef flank steak	All other pork
Fish canned in water	*Calf heart	Anything w/butter sauce
Lean ham	Lean lamb	Anything w/cream sauce
Lobster	*Liver	Anything with cheese
Other fish, not fried	Pork feet	Beef ribs
*Other organ meat	*Pork pancreas	Beef/pork tongue
Other seafood	Poultry, dark meat	Fried chicken/fried meat
Pork tenderloin, lean	Poultry with skin	Fried fish/fried seafood
Poultry, white w/gravy	Regular ham	Hamburger/meatloaf
Poultry, white w/o skin	Veal	Hot dog/sausage/kielbasa
Raw/steamed clams	Wild game	Other pork
Shrimp		Other steak/other beef
		Pork tail
*very high in cholesterol	*very high cholesterol	Poultry, dark w/skin

Calorie Light	Calorie Moderate	Calorie Dense
(9.0 ounces)	(6.0 ounces)	(4.0 ounces)
Bouillon (unlimited amt)	Soup, black bean	Soup, any chunky kind
Soup, beef mushroom	Soup, chicken dumpling	Soup, any made w/milk
Soup, beef noodle	Soup, cream of, w/water	Soup, bean w/bacon
Soup, chicken gumbo	Soup, pepper pot	Soup, bean w/franks
Soup, chicken noodle	Soup, tomato bisque	Soup, cheese
Soup, chicken vegetable	Soup, tomato with rice	Soup, chicken mushrm
Soup, chicken with rice		Soup, chili beef
Soup, Manh clam chowdr		Soup, N.E. clam chowdr
Soup, minestrone		Soup, pea green
Soup, mushrm w/barley		Soup, split pea w/ham
Soup, onion		Soup, tomato beef noodl
Soup, oyster stew w/watr		
Soup, Scotch broth		
Soup, tomato (w/water)		
Soup, turkey noodle		
Soup, turkey vegetable		
Soup, vegetable beef		
Soup, vegetarian vegetabl		

(6.5 ounces)	(4.0 ounces)	(1.5 ounce)
Fruit canned in juice	Bananas	Candied fruit
Fruit canned light syrup	Breadfruit	Coconut
Other fresh fruit	Crabapples	Dates
	Elderberries	Dried Fruit
	Fresh figs	Prunes
	Fruit canned hvy syrup	Raisins
	Passion fruit	
	Plantain	
	Sweetened fruit	

(15.0 ounces)	(8.5 ounces)	(5.0 ounces)
Cultured buttermilk	Chocolate milk	Eggnog
Low-fat milk	Coffee flavor milk	Hot cocoa made w/milk
Skim milk	Low-fat chocolate milk	Milk shake
	Whole goat milk	Whole sheep milk
	Whole milk	

DINNER -- Choose 1 item from each section. Select mostly "Light" foods.

Calorie Light	Calorie Moderate	Calorie Dense
(13.5 ounces)	(6.0 ounces)	(2.5 ounce)
Garden salad, no dressing	Salad with croutons	Any salad w/dressing
Salad with no-fat dressing	Salad with olives	Any salad w/mayonnaise
		Any salad with oil
		Chef salad/Caesar salad
(8.5 ounces)	(5.0 ounces)	(3.5 ounces)
Beef stew	Burritos	Cheese fondue
Casserole in tomato sauce	Chicken a la king	Chili con queso
Chili	Corned beef hash	Meatloaf
Diet entrees, except fried	Curry dishes with rice	Nachos
Pasta in tomato sauce	Enchiladas	Pasta in cream sauce
Shrimp creole	Macaroni and cheese	Pasta w/carbonara sauce
	Newburg dishes w/pasta	Stuffed potato skins
	Newburg dishes w/rice	Quiche
	Other casseroles	
	Other frozen entrees	
	Other pasta w/cheese	
	Other pasta w/meat	
	Pizza	
	Pot pies	
	Tacos	
	Tuna casserole	
(5.0 ounces)	(3.5 ounces)	(1.5 ounces)
Any rice/potato w/gravy	Any rice/potato w/butter	Any fried potatoes
Plain baked potato	Any rice/potato w/chees	Potato skins, baked/fried
Plain boiled potato	Baked potato, sour crm	
Plain brown rice	Beef flavored rice	
Plain white rice	Chicken flavored rice	
Scalloped potatoes	Chinese fried rice	
Spanish rice	Other flavored rice	

(13.5 ounces)	(6.5 ounces)	(3.5 ounces)
Asparagus	Acorn/butternut squash	Any deep fry veg(1.5 oz)
Bamboo shoots	Beets	Any veg w/butter, marg
Broccoli	Brussels sprouts	Any veg w/cheese sauce
Butterbur	Carrots	Arrowhead
Cauliflower	Hubbard/winter squash	Baked beans
Crookneck/scallop squash	Hyacinth beans	Broad beans
Eggplant	Kale	Corn/creamed corn
Rhubarb	Leeks	Green peas/cowpeas
Sauerkraut	Mixed vegetables	Kidney/pinto beans
Spaghetti/summer squash	Navy beans	Lima beans
Spinach	Okra	Parsnips
String beans	Onions	Pigeon peas
Fresh or stewed tomatoes	Rutabagas	Soybeans
Turnips	Shellie beans	Succotash
Zucchini	Winged beans	Sweet potatoes/yams

(6.5 ounces)	(2.5 ounce)	(1.5 ounce)
Fresh fruit	Frozen yogurt (4.0 oz)	Cake and pastry
Gelatin dessert	Fudgsicles	Candy and chocolate
Gelatin w/fruit	Ice milk	Cookies
Lo cal gelatin (unlimited)	Popsicles (4.0 ounces)	Ice cream/sundae
Lo cal popsicle (unlimit)	Pudding	Pie
Lo cal pudding	Sherbert	

DAILY MENU PLAN #10 -- 2000 Calories

BREAKFAST -- Choose 1 item from each section (i.e., choose 1 breakfast bread product, 1 cereal, and 1 fruit). Select mostly "Light" foods.

Calorie Light	Calorie Moderate	Calorie Dense
(3.5 ounces)	(2.5 ounces)	(2.0 ounce)
French toast with syrup	Bagel with cream cheese	Biscuits with butter
Pancakes with syrup	Brown & serve rolls	Croissant
Plain bagel, any type	Coffee cake	Croissant with butter
Plain cornbread, homemd	English muffin w/butter	Danish pastry
Plain English muffins	Muffins, any type	Donuts, any type
Plain toast, low calorie	Pancakes w/butter,syrup	Matzo with butter
Toast w/low cal spread	Plain biscuits	
Waffles with syrup	Sweet rolls	
	Toast w/butter and jelly	
	Waffles w/butter, syrup	
(13.0 ounces)	(1.5 ounces)	(1.5 ounce)
Cream of wheat, cooked	*Bran cereals	*Granola-type cereals
Grits, cooked	*Flakes w/dried fruit	*Sugar-coated cereals
Malt-o-meal, cooked	*Other cereals	*High-sugar cereals
Maypo, cooked	*Plain flakes, any type	
Oatmeal, any type,cooked	*Wheat squares w/fruit	
Other hot cereal, cooked		
Ralston, cooked		
Wheatena, cooked	*Plus skim milk (6.5 oz)	*Plus skim milk (6.5 oz)
(5.5 ounces)	(3.5 ounces)	(1.0 ounce)
Fruit canned in juice	Bananas	Candied fruit
Fruit canned in lt syrup	Breadfruit	Coconut
Other fresh fruit	Crabapples	Dates
	Elderberries	Dried fruit
	Fresh figs	Prunes
	Fruit canned hvy syrup	Raisins
	Passion fruit	
	Plantain	
	Sweetened fruit	

LUNCH -- Choose 1 item from each section. Select mostly "Light" foods.

Calorie Light	Calorie Moderate	Calorie Dense
(8.5 ounces)	(6.5 ounces)	(6.0 ounces)
Sndwch,91% fat-free meat	Sndwch, 82-92% fat-free	Any croissant sandwich
Sandwich, grilled fish	Sandwich, regular ham	Any fried sandwich
Sandwich, grilled chicken		Any sandwich w/bacon
Sandwich, tuna (in water)		Any sandwich w/cheese
Sandwich, turkey		Any sandwich w/mayo
Sandwich, turkey breast		Burger/hot dog, all types
Sndwch, vegetarn(13.5oz)		Sandwich, meatball
		Sandwich, other meat
		Sndwch, p.b. &/or jelly
		Sandwich, submarine
(13.5 ounces)	(6.0 ounces)	(2.5 ounce)
Garden salad, no dressing	Salad with croutons	Any salad w/dressing
Salad with no-fat dressing	Salad with olives	Any salad w/mayonnaise
		Any salad with oil
		Chef salad/Caesar salad
(8.5 ounces)	(6.0 ounces)	(1.5 ounce)
Apple cider	Apricot nectar	Coconut milk
Apple juice	Cranberry juice	
Blackberry juice	Cran-apple juice	
Grapefruit juice	Cran-apricot juice	
Grapefruit juice, sweetnd	Cran-grape juice	
Orange juice	Grape juice	
Orange-grapefruit juice	Orange-apricot juice	
Tangerine juice	Papaya nectar	
Tangelo juice	Passion fruit juice	
Tomato juice (16.5 oz)	Peach nectar	
	Pear nectar	
	Pineapple juice	
	Pineapple-grapefrt juice	
	Pineapple-orange juice	
	Pine-orange-banana juice	
	Prune juice	

(7.5 ounces)	(2.5 ounces)	(1.5 ounces)
Cottage cheese, any type	Feta cheese	All other cheese
Lite ricotta	Neufchatel cheese	
Frozen yogurt	Part-skim mozzarella	
Yogurt, any type	Ricotta cheese	
	Skim mozzarella cheese	

DINNER -- Choose 1 item from each section. Select mostly "Light" foods.

Calorie Light	Calorie Moderate	Calorie Dense
(13.5 ounces)	(6.0 ounces)	(2.5 ounces)
Garden salad, no dressing	Salad with croutons	Any salad w/dressing
Salad with no-fat dressing	Salad with olives	Any salad w/mayonnaise
		Any salad with oil
		Chef salad/Caesar salad
(6.5 ounces)	(5.0 ounces)	(3.5 ounces)
Any 91% fat-free meat	Any 82% fat-free meat	All other lunch meat
Crab	Beef flank steak	All other pork
Fish canned in water	*Calf heart	Anything w/butter sauce
Lean ham	Lean lamb	Anything w/cream sauce
Lobster	*Liver	Anything with cheese
Other fish, not fried	Pork feet	Beef ribs
*Other organ meat	*Pork pancreas	Beef/pork tongue
Other seafood	Poultry, dark meat	Fried chicken/fried meat
Pork tenderloin, lean	Poultry with skin	Fried fish/fried seafood
Poultry, white w/gravy	Regular ham	Hamburger/meatloaf
Poultry, white w/o skin	Veal	Hot dog/sausage/kielbasa
Raw/steamed clams	Wild game	Other pork
Shrimp		Other steak/other beef
		Pork tail
*very high in cholesterol	*very high cholesterol	Poultry, dark w/skin
(1.5 ounces)	(1.5 ounce)	(1.0 ounce)
Plain bagels, any type	Bagels w/cream cheese	All other crackers
Cornbread	Bread/rolls with butter	All other nuts
Plain muffins, any type	Croissants	Cheetos/cheese curls
Plain bread/rolls	Honey-coated grahams	Chex snack mix
Roasted chestnuts	Matzo/bread sticks	Chips, any variety
	Oyster crackers	Microwave popcorn
	Plain air-pop popcorn	Popcorn, oil popped
	Plain graham crackers	Popcorn with butter
	Pretzels	Seeds, any type
	Soda crackers	
	Triscuit crackers	

(13.5 ounces)	(6.5 ounces)	(3.5 ounces)
Asparagus	Acorn/butternut squash	Any deep fry veg(1.5 oz)
Bamboo shoots	Beets	Any veg w/butter, marg
Broccoli	Brussels sprouts	Any veg w/cheese sauce
Butterbur	Carrots	Arrowhead
Cauliflower	Hubbard/winter squash	Baked beans
Crookneck/scallop squash	Hyacinth beans	Broad beans
Eggplant	Kale	Corn/creamed corn
Rhubarb	Leeks	Green peas/cowpeas
Sauerkraut	Mixed vegetables	Kidney/pinto beans
Spaghetti/summer squash	Navy beans	Lima beans
Spinach	Okra	Parsnips
String beans	Onions	Pigeon peas
Fresh or stewed tomatoes	Rutabagas	Soybeans
Turnips	Shellie beans	Succotash
Zucchini	Winged beans	Sweet potatoes/yams

(6.5 ounces)	(2.5 ounces)	(1.5 ounce)
Fresh fruit	Frozen yogurt (4.0 oz)	Cake and pastry
Gelatin dessert	Fudgsicles	Candy and chocolate
Gelatin w/fruit	Ice milk	Cookies
Lo cal gelatin (unlimited)	Popsicles (4.0 ounces)	Ice cream/sundae
Lo cal popsicle (unlimit)	Pudding	Pie
Lo cal pudding	Sherbert	

EXERCISE GRAPHS

Whether your goal is to lose weight or simply keep from gaining weight, sensible exercise is extremely beneficial. As explained earlier, in order to lose 1 pound of body weight, you must expend 3500 calories more than you consume. With even moderate exercise, over a period of time, the number of calories expended is significant. For example, if you weigh 180 pounds and you exercise moderately for one hour per exercise session, three times per week, the graph at the bottom of page 73 indicates that you will lose approximately 1/2 pound per week. If your exercise is heavy rather than moderate, the graph shows that you will lose approximately 1 pound per week.

In addition to the direct effects of exercise on weight loss, there is an extra bonus. Exercise speeds your metabolism not only during the activity but for some time afterwards. The extent of this extra bonus varies from person to person. Also, when you exercise, you promote weight loss in the form of fat rather than muscle. (For more information on exercise, see pages 9 and 10 of the Nutrition and Exercise Guidelines chapter.)

The graphs on pages 68 through 81 will enable you to see both the approximate number of calories used during your exercise sessions and the weight loss attributable to your exercise. The graphs are designed for people who weigh 100 pounds to 300 pounds. Make sure that you use the graph that most accurately approximates your body weight.

Before using any of the graphs, you must first categorize your exercise as light, moderate or heavy. The classifications of exercise intensity listed on the next page were used in creating the graphs, and they should serve as a guide for categorizing your own physical activity.

Please note: If your activities or exercises appear to be between classifications, then literally read between the lines when viewing the graphs. Also, please note that if you have more than one exercise, the effect on calories used and weight loss is cumulative; simply add the individual exercises to arrive at the total result.

Light Intensity Exercise

Bicycling (6-8 mph)
Bowling
Golf (without cart)
Ice/roller skating (5 mph)
Light calisthenics
Rowing (light)
Tennis (doubles)
Volleyball (noncompetitive)
Walking (3-4 mph)

Moderate Intensity Exercise

Bicycling (12 mph)
Cross-country skiing (slow)
Low impact aerobics
Racket sports (noncompetitive)
Ice/roller skating (10 mph)
Rowing (18 strokes per minute)
Running (6-7 mph)
Swimming (2 mph)
Walking (5 mph)
Water skiing/downhill skiing
Weight lifting (circuit)

Heavy Intensity Exercise

Basketball
Bicycling (20 mph)
Climbing stairs (100 per minute)
Cross-country skiing (vigorous)
High-impact/step aerobics
Hockey (competitive)
Racket sports (competitive)
Rowing (30 strokes per minute)
Running (8-10 mph)
Soccer (competitive)
Swimming (2.5 mph)

Calories Used in Exercise

Body Weight 100 - 120 lbs.

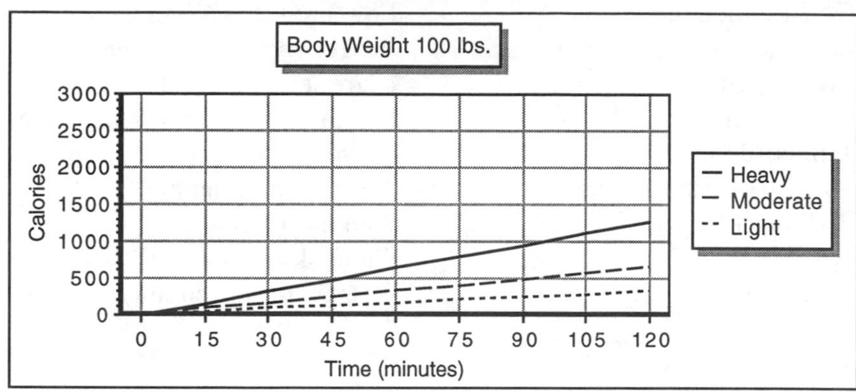

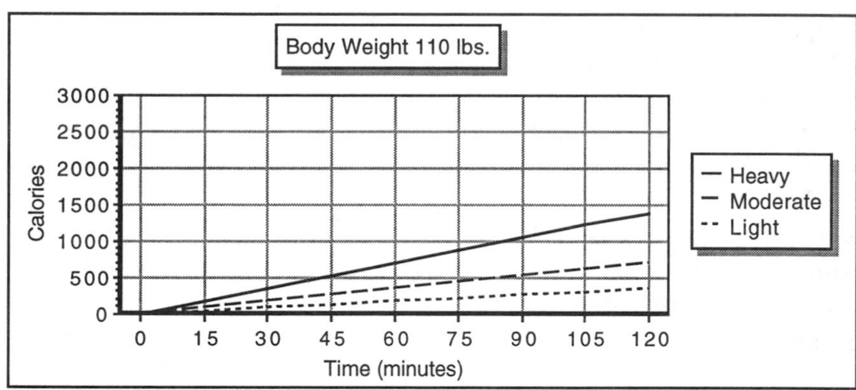

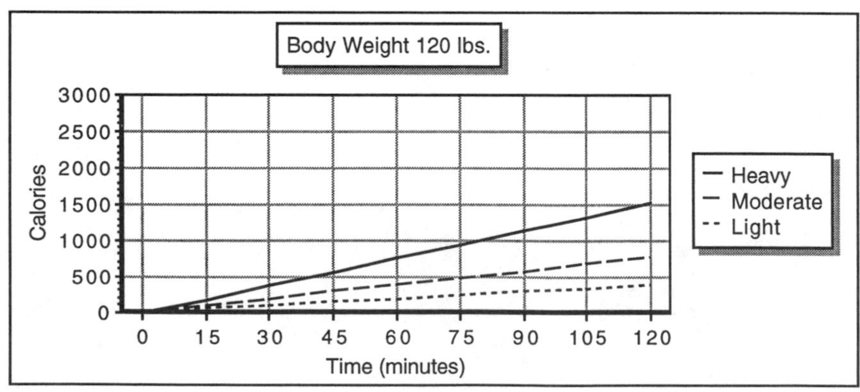

Weight Loss from Exercise

Body Weight 100 - 120 lbs.

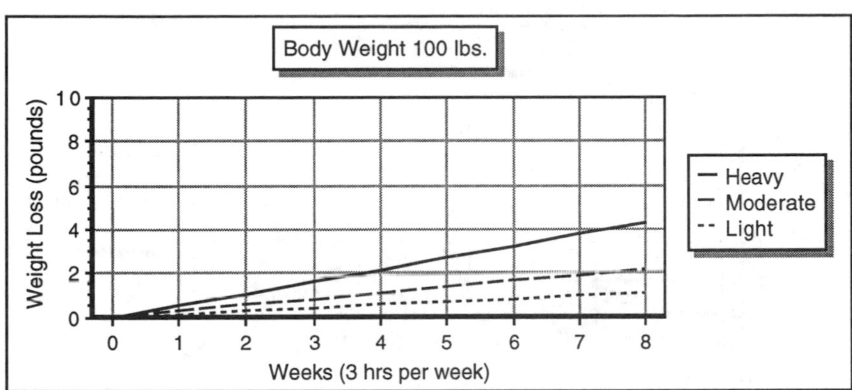

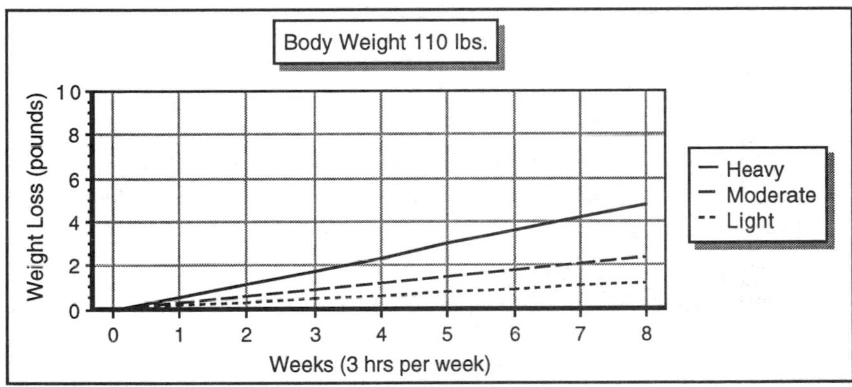

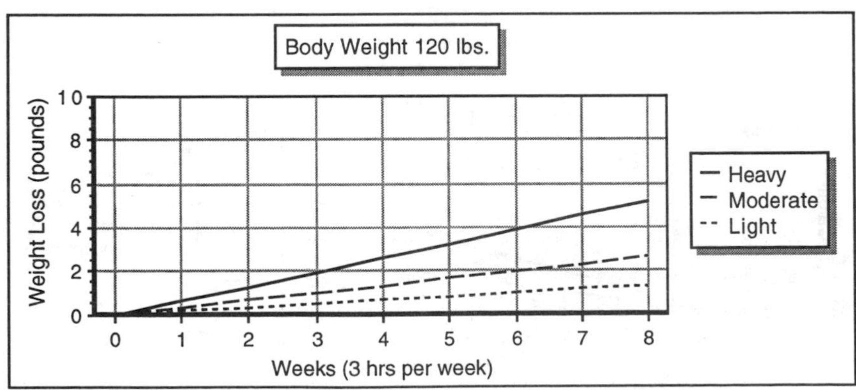

Calories Used in Exercise

Body Weight 130 - 150 lbs.

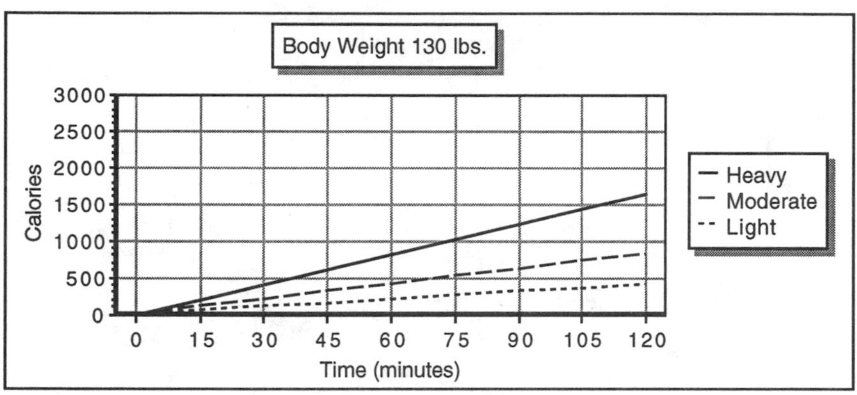

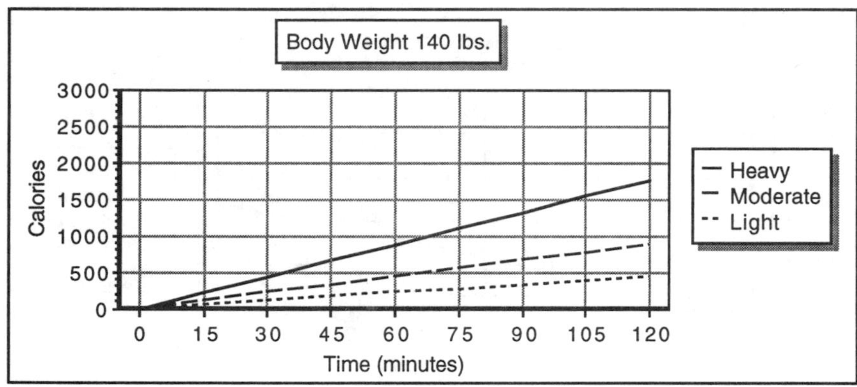

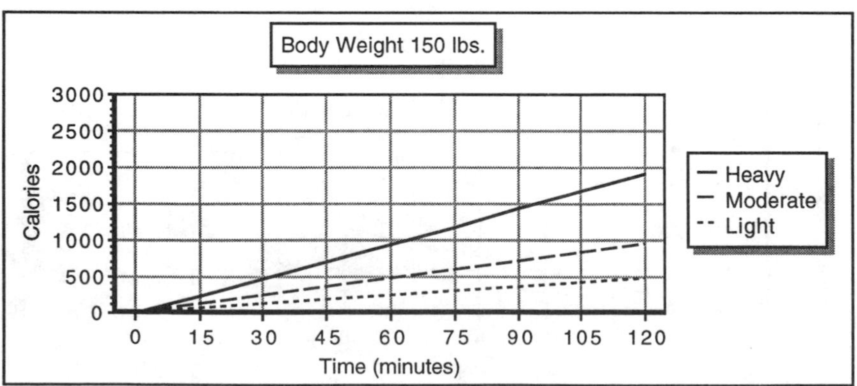

Weight Loss from Exercise

Body Weight 130 - 150 lbs.

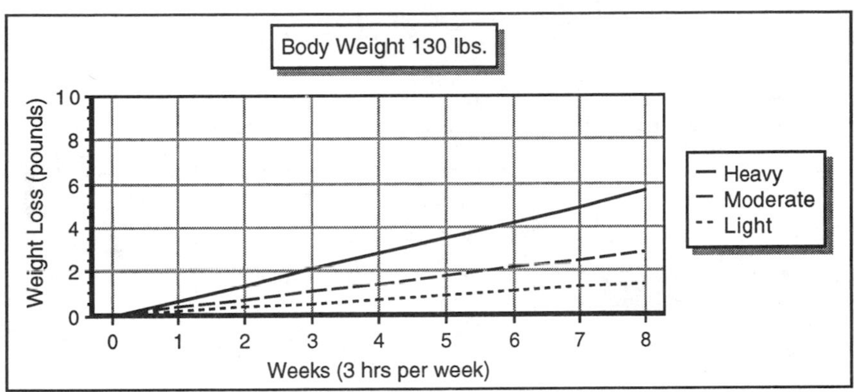

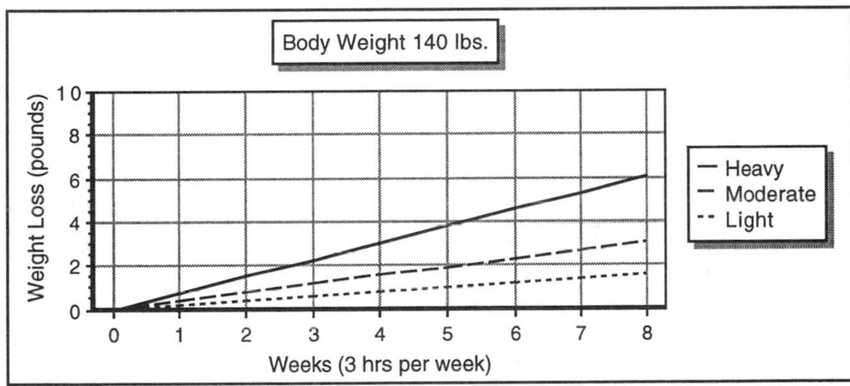

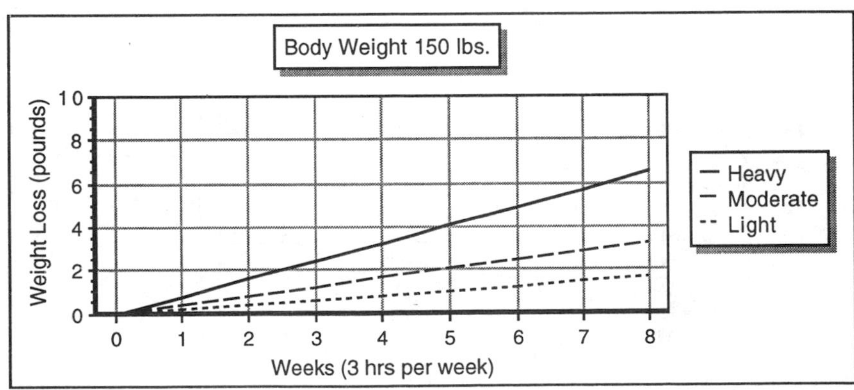

Calories Used in Exercise

Body Weight 160 - 180 lbs.

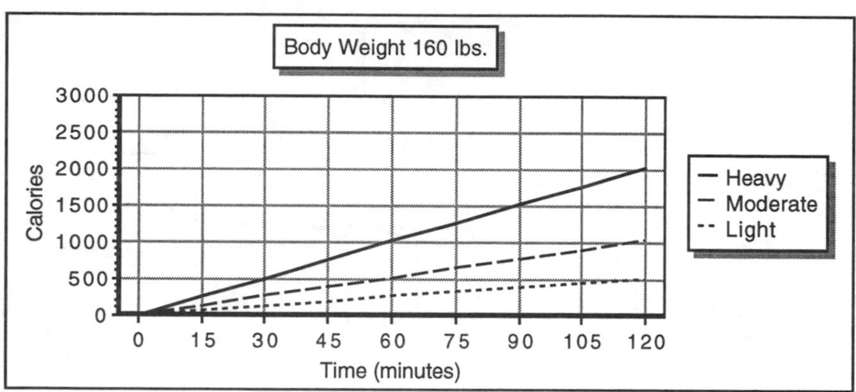

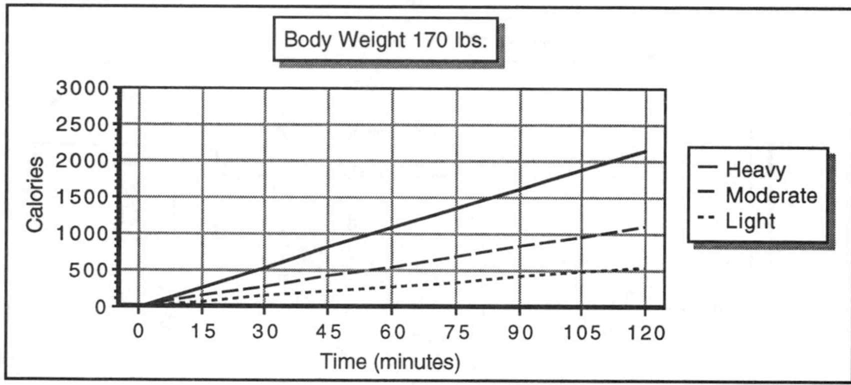

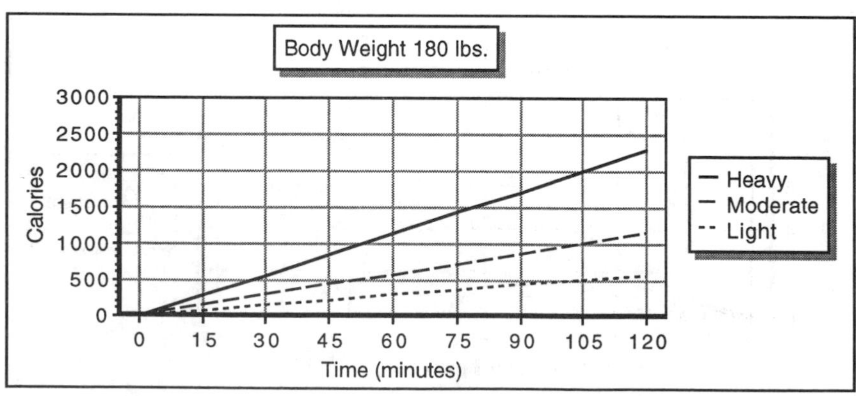

Weight Loss from Exercise

Body Weight 160 - 180 lbs.

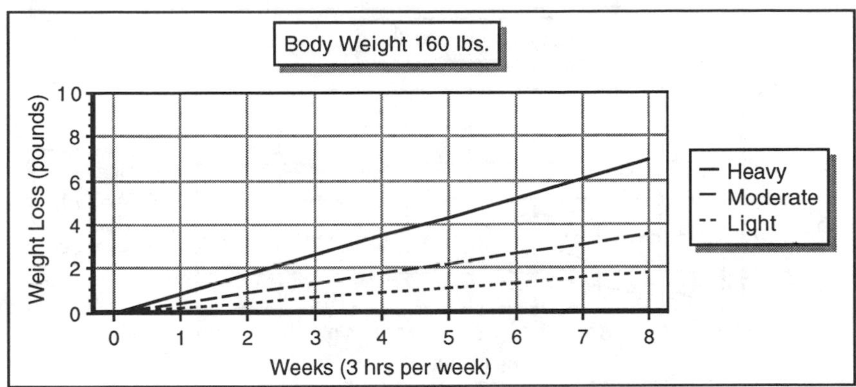

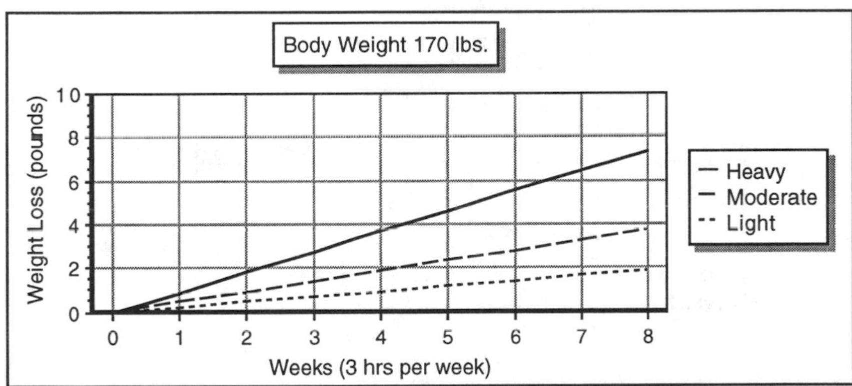

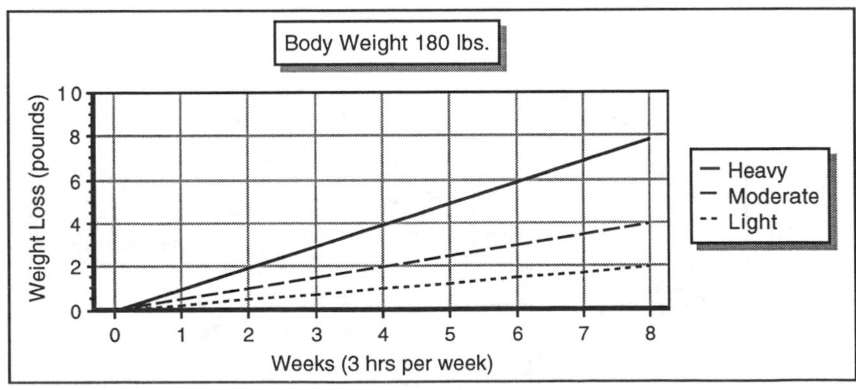

Calories Used in Exercise

Body Weight 190 - 210 lbs.

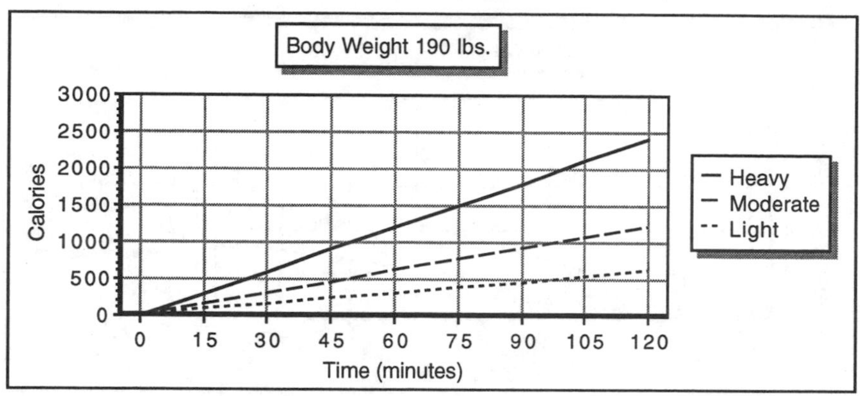

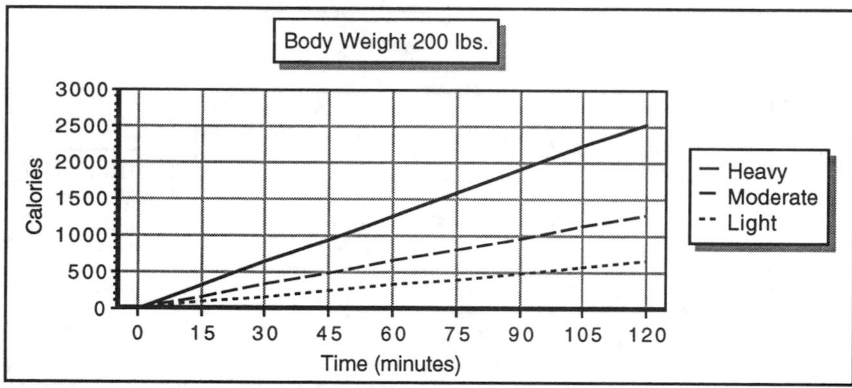

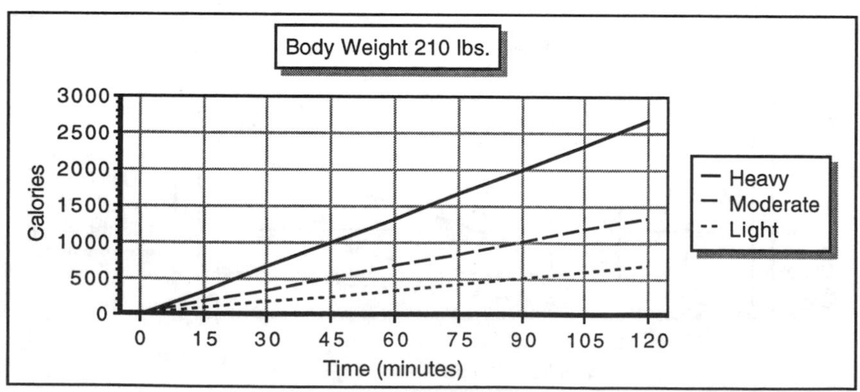

Weight Loss from Exercise

Body Weight 190 - 210 lbs.

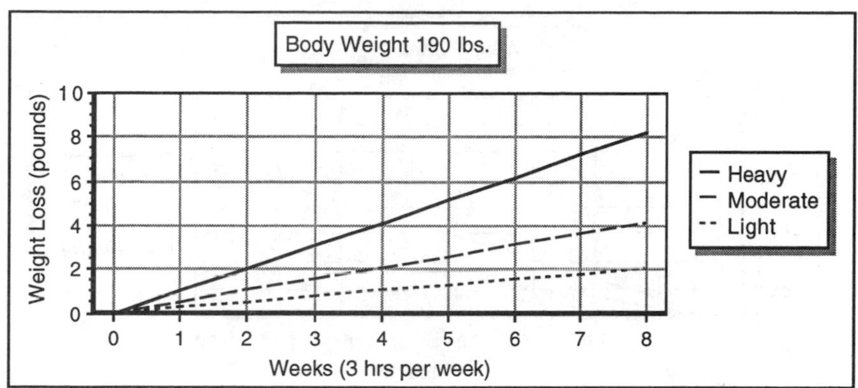

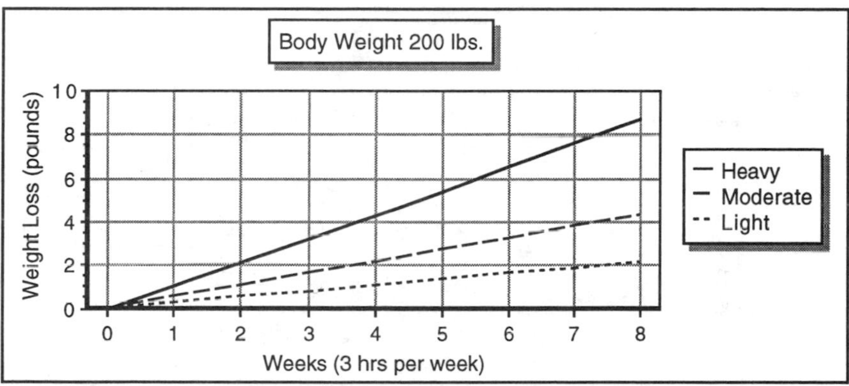

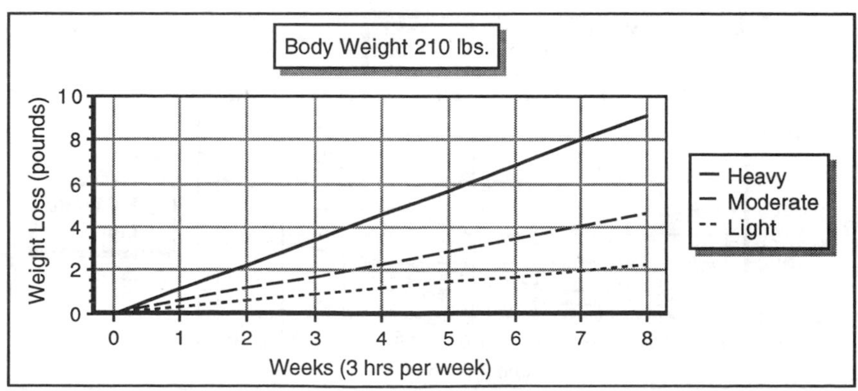

Calories Used in Exercise

Body Weight 220 - 240 lbs.

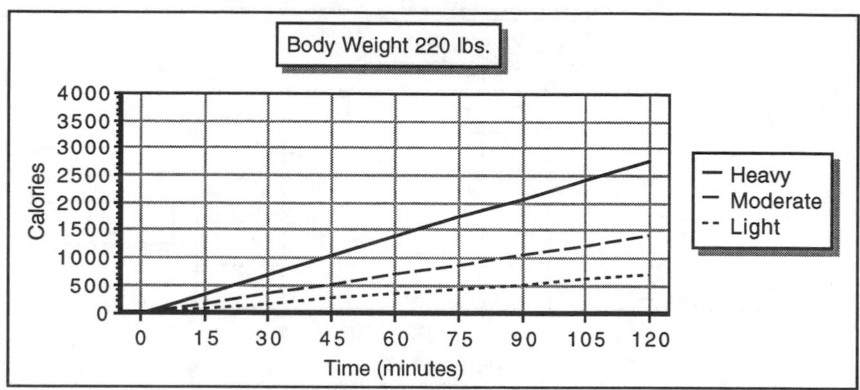

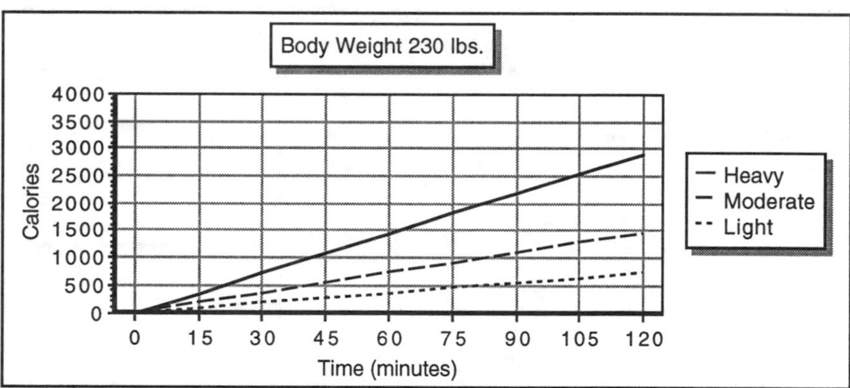

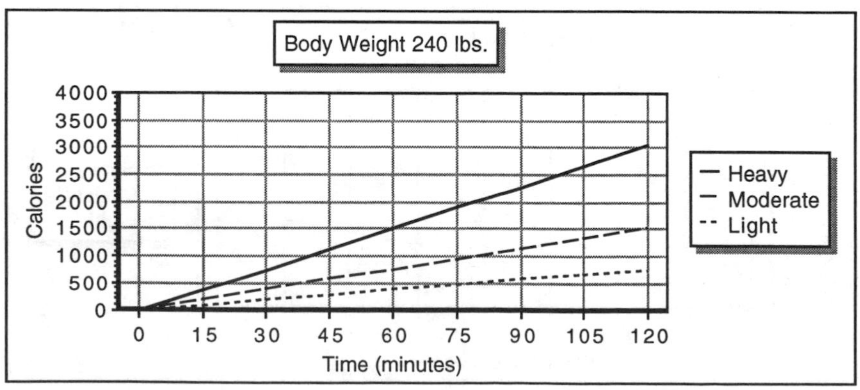

Weight Loss from Exercise

Body Weight 220 - 240 lbs.

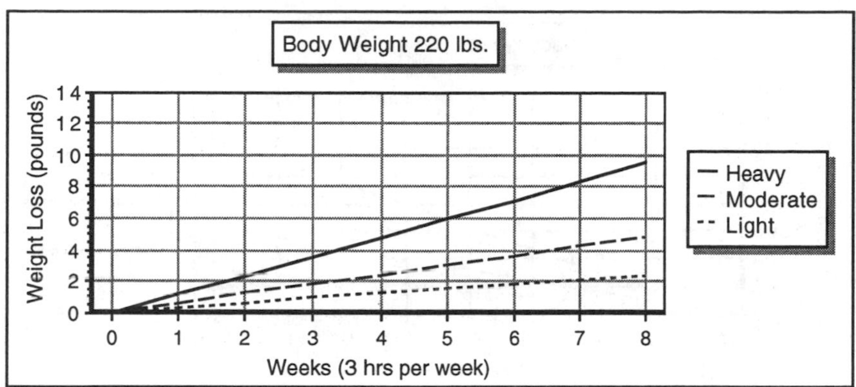

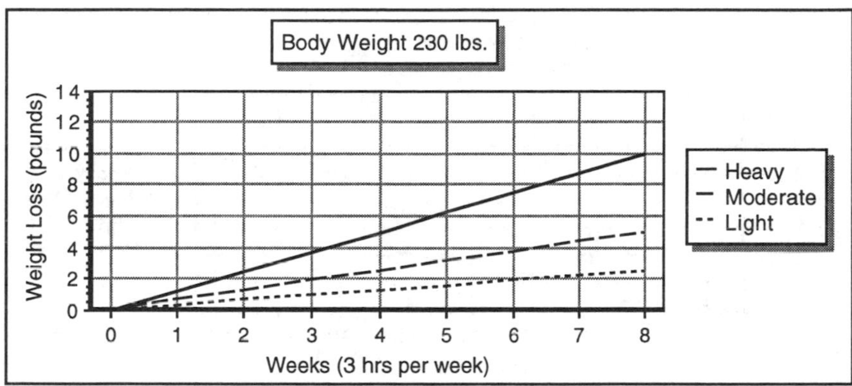

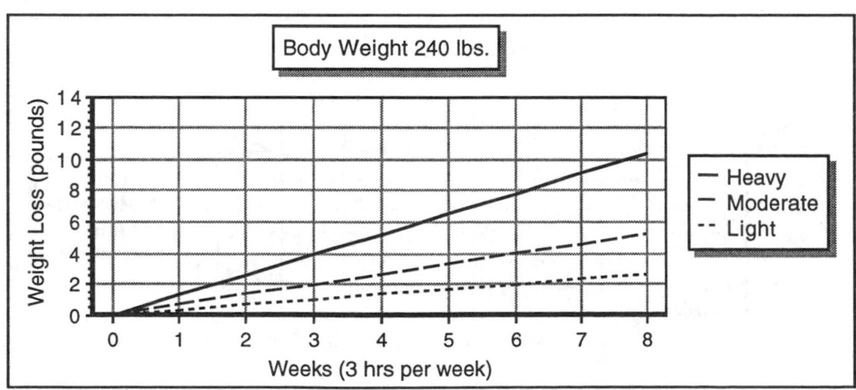

Calories Used in Exercise

Body Weight 250 - 270 lbs.

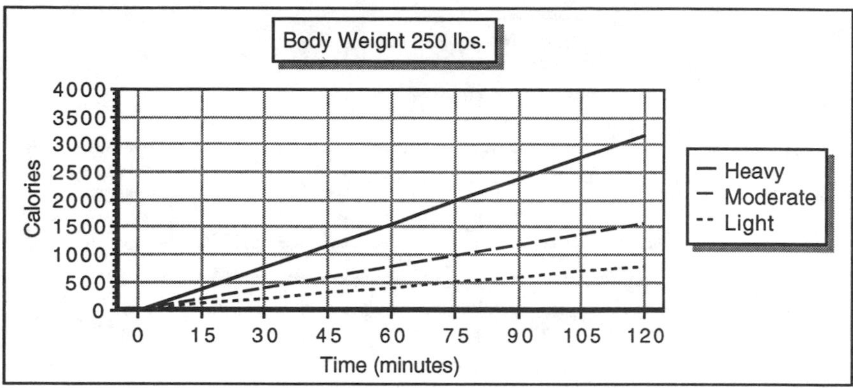

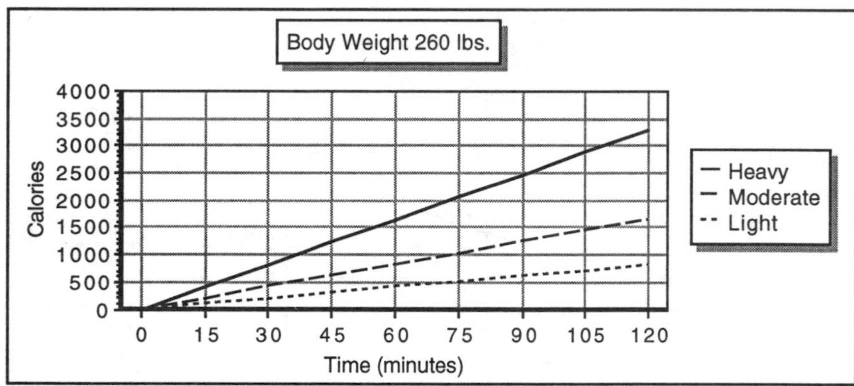

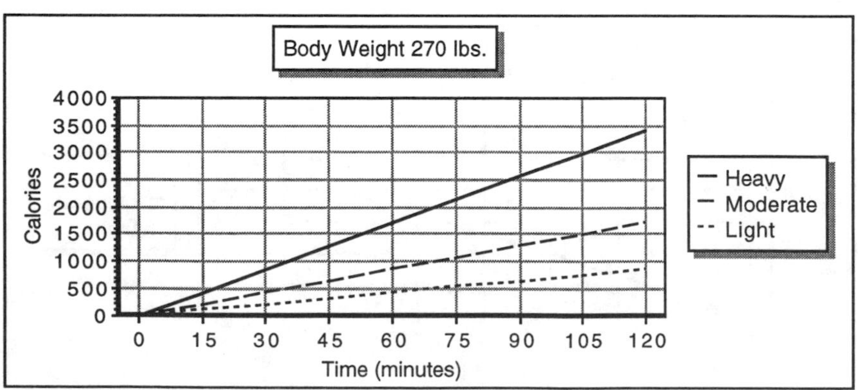

Weight Loss from Exercise

Body Weight 250 - 270 lbs.

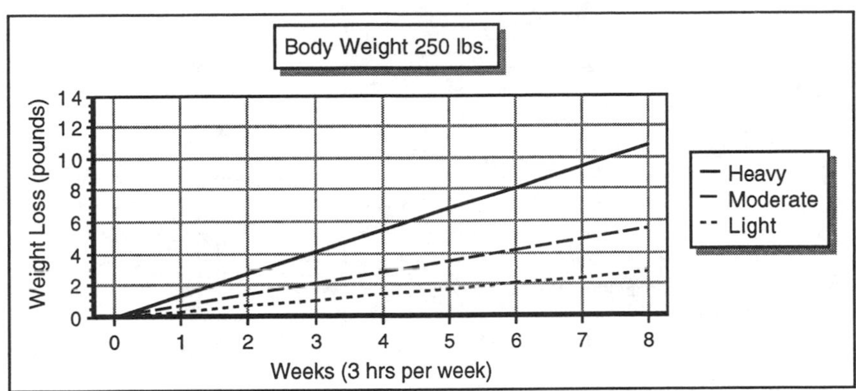

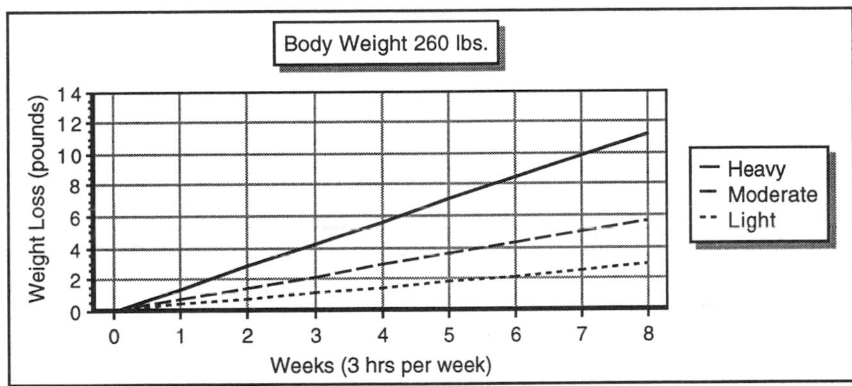

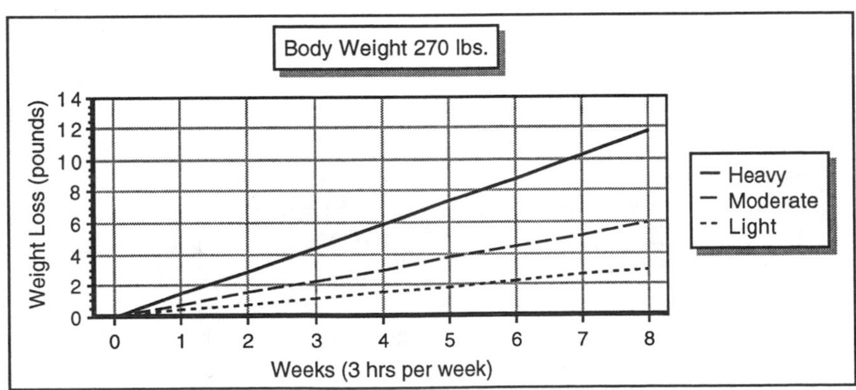

Calories Used in Exercise

Body Weight 280 - 300 lbs.

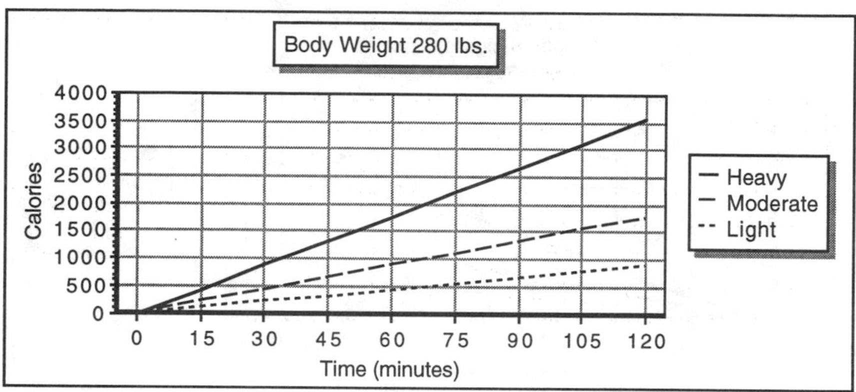

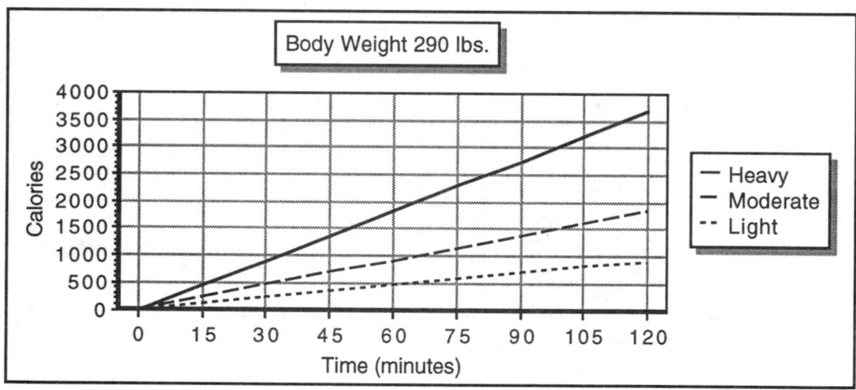

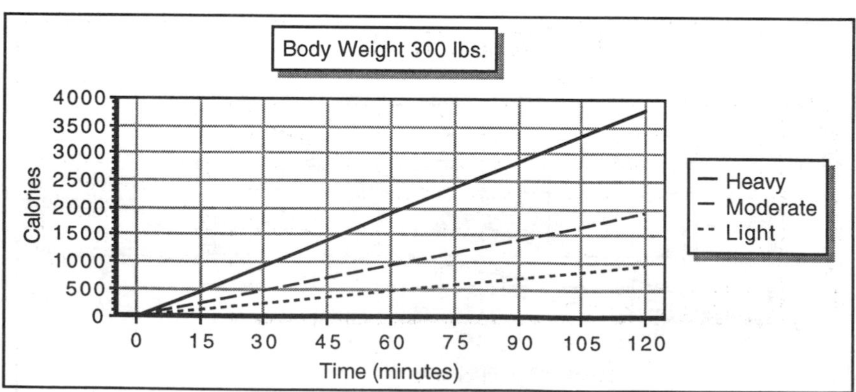

Weight Loss from Exercise

Body Weight 280 - 300 lbs.

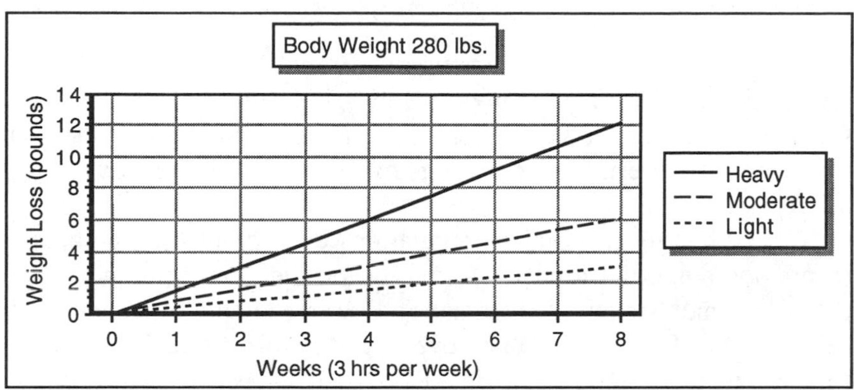

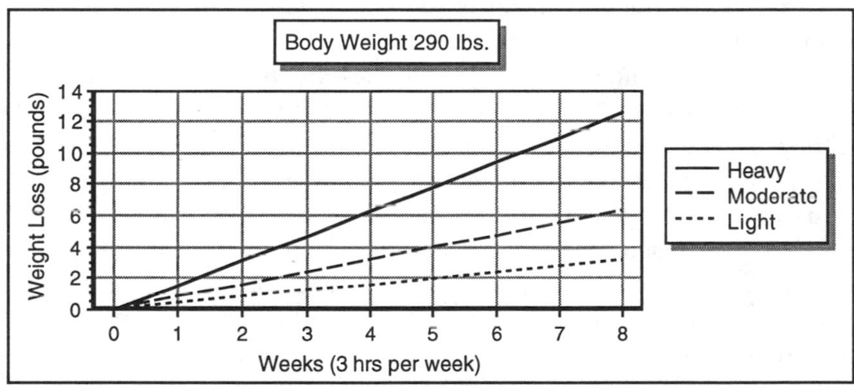

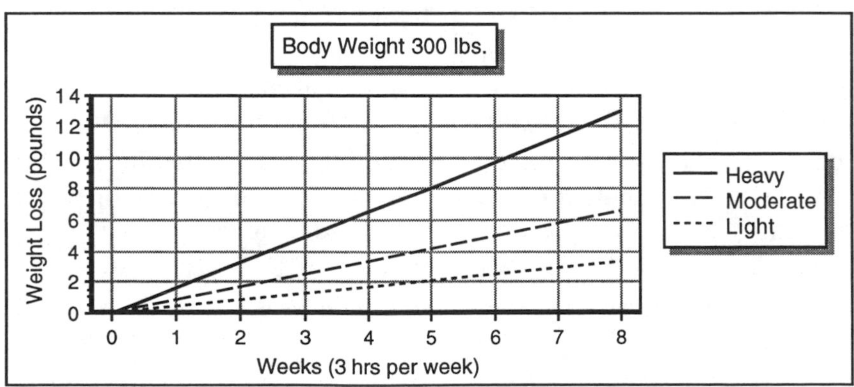

SHOPPERS' GUIDELINES

The purpose of the Shoppers' Guidelines is to provide you with a simple tool for buying low-fat foods. The Shoppers' Guidelines will enable you to determine, at a glance, whether the foods you are considering purchasing have the level of fat that is appropriate for you.

Although government regulations do require food companies to provide some nutritional information on their food product labels, the government-required information does not include percentage of calories from fat. Instead, the government requires a listing of the fat percentage of RDA per serving based on an average daily caloric intake. As a result, a government-approved food label may indicate that a food is not a significant source of fat, even if 100% of its calories comes from fat!

You will note that our guidelines are listed in increments of 5%, starting at 5% and continuing through 50%. To use the Shoppers' Guidelines, first decide which guideline you wish to follow. The specific determination of which guideline is most appropriate for you should be made with the help of your physician or registered/licensed dietitian. After you have made the appropriate determination, go to the page that contains the guideline that you need. (You may wish to photocopy the guideline so that you can take it with you to the grocery store.) Each guideline has two rows of numbers: the first is the total number of calories, and the second is the grams of fat. To use the guideline, select any food product that has a label and look on the label for the total number of calories. After you have located that number, find it in the first column of your guideline. Then look to the right of that number for the corresponding grams of fat. Once you have identified that number, look on the label of the food product to see whether the food contains less than that number; if not, then the food does not meet your guideline, and you may want to purchase something else.

SHOPPERS' GUIDELINE -- 5% Fat

This table lists grams of fat which total 5 percent of calories. To use this table, look at a food label and find the number of calories per serving. Then find the corresponding number in the calories column of this guide which is closest to the number of calories on the product label. Now look to the next column in the same row, and you will find the number of grams of fat equal to 5 percent of calories.

Calories	Fat (g)	Calories	Fat (g)	Calories	Fat (g)
5	-----> 0.0	155	-----> 0.9	305	-----> 1.7
10	-----> 0.1	160	-----> 0.9	310	-----> 1.7
15	-----> 0.1	165	-----> 0.9	315	-----> 1.7
20	-----> 0.1	170	-----> 0.9	320	-----> 1.8
25	-----> 0.1	175	-----> 1.0	325	-----> 1.8
30	-----> 0.2	180	-----> 1.0	330	-----> 1.8
35	-----> 0.2	185	-----> 1.0	335	-----> 1.9
40	-----> 0.2	190	-----> 1.1	340	-----> 1.9
45	-----> 0.2	195	-----> 1.1	345	-----> 1.9
50	-----> 0.3	200	-----> 1.1	350	-----> 1.9
55	-----> 0.3	205	-----> 1.1	355	-----> 2.0
60	-----> 0.3	210	-----> 1.2	360	-----> 2.0
65	-----> 0.4	215	-----> 1.2	365	-----> 2.0
70	-----> 0.4	220	-----> 1.2	370	-----> 2.1
75	-----> 0.4	225	-----> 1.2	375	-----> 2.1
80	-----> 0.4	230	-----> 1.3	380	-----> 2.1
85	-----> 0.5	235	-----> 1.3	385	-----> 2.1
90	-----> 0.5	240	-----> 1.3	390	-----> 2.2
95	-----> 0.5	245	-----> 1.4	395	-----> 2.2
100	-----> 0.6	250	-----> 1.4	400	-----> 2.2
105	-----> 0.6	255	-----> 1.4	405	-----> 2.2
110	-----> 0.6	260	-----> 1.4	410	-----> 2.3
115	-----> 0.6	265	-----> 1.5	415	-----> 2.3
120	-----> 0.7	270	-----> 1.5	420	-----> 2.3
125	-----> 0.7	275	-----> 1.5	425	-----> 2.4
130	-----> 0.7	280	-----> 1.6	430	-----> 2.4
135	-----> 0.7	285	-----> 1.6	435	-----> 2.4
140	-----> 0.8	290	-----> 1.6	440	-----> 2.4
145	-----> 0.8	295	-----> 1.6	445	-----> 2.5
150	-----> 0.8	300	-----> 1.7	450	-----> 2.5

SHOPPERS' GUIDELINE -- 10% Fat

This table lists grams of fat which total 10 percent of calories. To use this table, look at a food label and find the number of calories per serving. Then find the corresponding number in the calories column of this guide which is closest to the number of calories on the product label. Now look to the next column in the same row, and you will find the number of grams of fat equal to 10 percent of calories.

Calories	Fat (g)	Calories	Fat (g)	Calories	Fat (g)
5	-----> 0.1	155	-----> 1.7	305	-----> 3.3
10	-----> 0.1	160	-----> 1.8	310	-----> 3.4
15	-----> 0.2	165	-----> 1.8	315	-----> 3.5
20	-----> 0.2	170	-----> 1.9	320	-----> 3.5
25	-----> 0.3	175	-----> 1.9	325	-----> 3.6
30	-----> 0.3	180	-----> 2.0	330	-----> 3.6
35	-----> 0.4	185	-----> 2.1	335	-----> 3.7
40	-----> 0.4	190	-----> 2.1	340	-----> 3.7
45	-----> 0.5	195	-----> 2.2	345	-----> 3.8
50	-----> 0.6	200	-----> 2.2	350	-----> 3.8
55	-----> 0.6	205	-----> 2.3	355	-----> 3.9
60	-----> 0.7	210	-----> 2.3	360	-----> 4.0
65	-----> 0.7	215	-----> 2.4	365	-----> 4.0
70	-----> 0.8	220	-----> 2.4	370	-----> 4.1
75	-----> 0.8	225	-----> 2.5	375	-----> 4.1
80	-----> 0.9	230	-----> 2.5	380	-----> 4.2
85	-----> 0.9	235	-----> 2.6	385	-----> 4.2
90	-----> 1.0	240	-----> 2.6	390	-----> 4.3
95	-----> 1.1	245	-----> 2.7	395	-----> 4.3
100	-----> 1.1	250	-----> 2.7	400	-----> 4.4
105	-----> 1.2	255	-----> 2.8	405	-----> 4.5
110	-----> 1.2	260	-----> 2.8	410	-----> 4.5
115	-----> 1.3	265	-----> 2.9	415	-----> 4.6
120	-----> 1.3	270	-----> 3.0	420	-----> 4.6
125	-----> 1.4	275	-----> 3.0	425	-----> 4.7
130	-----> 1.4	280	-----> 3.1	430	-----> 4.7
135	-----> 1.5	285	-----> 3.1	435	-----> 4.8
140	-----> 1.6	290	-----> 3.2	440	-----> 4.8
145	-----> 1.6	295	-----> 3.2	445	-----> 4.9
150	-----> 1.7	300	-----> 3.3	450	-----> 5.0

SHOPPERS' GUIDELINE -- 15% Fat

This table lists grams of fat which total 15 percent of calories. To use this table, look at a food label and find the number of calories per serving. Then find the corresponding number in the calories column of this guide which is closest to the number of calories on the product label. Now look to the next column in the same row, and you will find the number of grams of fat equal to 15 percent of calories.

Calories	Fat (g)	Calories	Fat (g)	Calories	Fat (g)
5	-----> 0.1	155	-----> 2.6	305	-----> 5.0
10	-----> 0.2	160	-----> 2.7	310	-----> 5.1
15	-----> 0.3	165	-----> 2.8	315	-----> 5.2
20	-----> 0.3	170	-----> 2.8	320	-----> 5.3
25	-----> 0.4	175	-----> 2.9	325	-----> 5.4
30	-----> 0.5	180	-----> 3.0	330	-----> 5.5
35	-----> 0.6	185	-----> 3.1	335	-----> 5.5
40	-----> 0.7	190	-----> 3.2	340	-----> 5.6
45	-----> 0.8	195	-----> 3.3	345	-----> 5.7
50	-----> 0.8	200	-----> 3.3	350	-----> 5.8
55	-----> 0.9	205	-----> 3.4	355	-----> 5.9
60	-----> 1.0	210	-----> 3.5	360	-----> 6.0
65	-----> 1.1	215	-----> 3.6	365	-----> 6.0
70	-----> 1.2	220	-----> 3.7	370	-----> 6.1
75	-----> 1.3	225	-----> 3.8	375	-----> 6.2
80	-----> 1.3	230	-----> 3.8	380	-----> 6.3
85	-----> 1.4	235	-----> 3.9	385	-----> 6.4
90	-----> 1.5	240	-----> 4.0	390	-----> 6.5
95	-----> 1.6	245	-----> 4.0	395	-----> 6.5
100	-----> 1.7	250	-----> 4.1	400	-----> 6.6
105	-----> 1.8	255	-----> 4.2	405	-----> 6.7
110	-----> 1.8	260	-----> 4.3	410	-----> 6.8
115	-----> 1.9	265	-----> 4.4	415	-----> 6.9
120	-----> 2.0	270	-----> 4.5	420	-----> 7.0
125	-----> 2.1	275	-----> 4.5	425	-----> 7.0
130	-----> 2.2	280	-----> 4.6	430	-----> 7.1
135	-----> 2.3	285	-----> 4.7	435	-----> 7.2
140	-----> 2.3	290	-----> 4.8	440	-----> 7.3
145	-----> 2.4	295	-----> 4.9	445	-----> 7.4
150	-----> 2.5	300	-----> 5.0	450	-----> 7.5

SHOPPERS' GUIDELINE -- 20% Fat

This table lists grams of fat which total 20 percent of calories. To use this table, look at a food label and find the number of calories per serving. Then find the corresponding number in the calories column of this guide which is closest to the number of calories on the product label. Now look to the next column in the same row, and you will find the number of grams of fat equal to 20 percent of calories.

Calories	Fat (g)	Calories	Fat (g)	Calories	Fat (g)
5	-----> 0.1	155	-----> 3.4	305	-----> 6.7
10	-----> 0.2	160	-----> 3.6	310	-----> 6.8
15	-----> 0.3	165	-----> 3.7	315	-----> 7.0
20	-----> 0.4	170	-----> 3.8	320	-----> 7.1
25	-----> 0.6	175	-----> 3.9	325	-----> 7.2
30	-----> 0.7	180	-----> 4.0	330	-----> 7.3
35	-----> 0.8	185	-----> 4.1	335	-----> 7.4
40	-----> 0.9	190	-----> 4.2	340	-----> 7.5
45	-----> 1.0	195	-----> 4.3	345	-----> 7.6
50	-----> 1.1	200	-----> 4.4	350	-----> 7.7
55	-----> 1.2	205	-----> 4.6	355	-----> 7.8
60	-----> 1.3	210	-----> 4.7	360	-----> 8.0
65	-----> 1.4	215	-----> 4.8	365	-----> 8.1
70	-----> 1.6	220	-----> 4.9	370	-----> 8.2
75	-----> 1.7	225	-----> 5.0	375	-----> 8.3
80	-----> 1.8	230	-----> 5.1	380	-----> 8.4
85	-----> 1.9	235	-----> 5.2	385	-----> 8.5
90	-----> 2.0	240	-----> 5.3	390	-----> 8.6
95	-----> 2.1	245	-----> 5.4	395	-----> 8.7
100	-----> 2.2	250	-----> 5.5	400	-----> 8.8
105	-----> 2.3	255	-----> 5.6	405	-----> 9.0
110	-----> 2.4	260	-----> 5.7	410	-----> 9.1
115	-----> 2.6	265	-----> 5.8	415	-----> 9.2
120	-----> 2.7	270	-----> 6.0	420	-----> 9.3
125	-----> 2.8	275	-----> 6.1	425	-----> 9.4
130	-----> 2.9	280	-----> 6.2	430	-----> 9.5
135	-----> 3.0	285	-----> 6.3	435	-----> 9.6
140	-----> 3.1	290	-----> 6.4	440	-----> 9.7
145	-----> 3.2	295	-----> 6.5	445	-----> 9.8
150	-----> 3.3	300	-----> 6.6	450	-----> 10.0

SHOPPERS' GUIDELINE -- 25% Fat

This table lists grams of fat which total 25 percent of calories. To use this table, look at a food label and find the number of calories per serving. Then find the corresponding number in the calories column of this guide which is closest to the number of calories on the product label. Now look to the next column in the same row, and you will find the number of grams of fat equal to 25 percent of calories.

Calories	Fat (g)	Calories	Fat (g)	Calories	Fat (g)
5	-----> 0.1	155	-----> 4.3	305	-----> 8.4
10	-----> 0.3	160	-----> 4.4	310	-----> 8.6
15	-----> 0.4	165	-----> 4.6	315	-----> 8.7
20	-----> 0.6	170	-----> 4.7	320	-----> 8.8
25	-----> 0.7	175	-----> 4.9	325	-----> 9.0
30	-----> 0.8	180	-----> 5.0	330	-----> 9.1
35	-----> 1.0	185	-----> 5.1	335	-----> 9.3
40	-----> 1.1	190	-----> 5.3	340	-----> 9.4
45	-----> 1.3	195	-----> 5.4	345	-----> 9.5
50	-----> 1.4	200	-----> 5.6	350	-----> 9.7
55	-----> 1.5	205	-----> 5.7	355	-----> 9.8
60	-----> 1.7	210	-----> 5.8	360	-----> 10.0
65	-----> 1.8	215	-----> 6.0	365	-----> 10.1
70	-----> 1.9	220	-----> 6.1	370	-----> 10.2
75	-----> 2.1	225	-----> 6.3	375	-----> 10.4
80	-----> 2.2	230	-----> 6.3	380	-----> 10.5
85	-----> 2.4	235	-----> 6.5	385	-----> 10.6
90	-----> 2.5	240	-----> 6.6	390	-----> 10.8
95	-----> 2.6	245	-----> 6.8	395	-----> 10.9
100	-----> 2.8	250	-----> 6.9	400	-----> 11.1
105	-----> 2.9	255	-----> 7.0	405	-----> 11.2
110	-----> 3.1	260	-----> 7.2	410	-----> 11.3
115	-----> 3.2	265	-----> 7.3	415	-----> 11.5
120	-----> 3.3	270	-----> 7.5	420	-----> 11.6
125	-----> 3.5	275	-----> 7.6	425	-----> 11.8
130	-----> 3.6	280	-----> 7.7	430	-----> 11.9
135	-----> 3.8	285	-----> 7.9	435	-----> 12.0
140	-----> 3.9	290	-----> 8.0	440	-----> 12.2
145	-----> 4.0	295	-----> 8.1	445	-----> 12.3
150	-----> 4.2	300	-----> 8.3	450	-----> 12.5

SHOPPERS' GUIDELINE -- 30% Fat

This table lists grams of fat which total 30 percent of calories. To use this table, look at a food label and find the number of calories per serving. Then find the corresponding number in the calories column of this guide which is closest to the number of calories on the product label. Now look to the next column in the same row, and you will find the number of grams of fat equal to 30 percent of calories.

Calories	Fat (g)	Calories	Fat (g)	Calories	Fat (g)
5	-----> 0.2	155	-----> 5.2	305	-----> 10.1
10	-----> 0.3	160	-----> 5.3	310	-----> 10.3
15	-----> 0.5	165	-----> 5.5	315	-----> 10.5
20	-----> 0.7	170	-----> 5.7	320	-----> 10.6
25	-----> 0.8	175	-----> 5.8	325	-----> 10.8
30	-----> 1.0	180	-----> 6.0	330	-----> 11.0
35	-----> 1.2	185	-----> 6.2	335	-----> 11.1
40	-----> 1.3	190	-----> 6.3	340	-----> 11.3
45	-----> 1.5	195	-----> 6.5	345	-----> 11.5
50	-----> 1.7	200	-----> 6.7	350	-----> 11.6
55	-----> 1.8	205	-----> 6.8	355	-----> 11.8
60	-----> 2.0	210	-----> 7.0	360	-----> 12.0
65	-----> 2.2	215	-----> 7.2	365	-----> 12.1
70	-----> 2.3	220	-----> 7.3	370	-----> 12.3
75	-----> 2.5	225	-----> 7.5	375	-----> 12.5
80	-----> 2.7	230	-----> 7.6	380	-----> 12.6
85	-----> 2.8	235	-----> 7.8	385	-----> 12.8
90	-----> 3.0	240	-----> 8.0	390	-----> 13.0
95	-----> 3.2	245	-----> 8.1	395	-----> 13.1
100	-----> 3.3	250	-----> 8.3	400	-----> 13.3
105	-----> 3.5	255	-----> 8.5	405	-----> 13.5
110	-----> 3.7	260	-----> 8.6	410	-----> 13.6
115	-----> 3.8	265	-----> 8.8	415	-----> 13.8
120	-----> 4.0	270	-----> 9.0	420	-----> 14.0
125	-----> 4.2	275	-----> 9.1	425	-----> 14.1
130	-----> 4.3	280	-----> 9.3	430	-----> 14.3
135	-----> 4.5	285	-----> 9.5	435	-----> 14.5
140	-----> 4.7	290	-----> 9.6	440	-----> 14.6
145	-----> 4.8	295	-----> 9.8	445	-----> 14.8
150	-----> 5.0	300	-----> 10.0	450	-----> 15.0

SHOPPERS' GUIDELINE -- 35% Fat

This table lists grams of fat which total 35 percent of calories. To use this table, look at a food label and find the number of calories per serving. Then find the corresponding number in the calories column of this guide which is closest to the number of calories on the product label. Now look to the next column in the same row, and you will find the number of grams of fat equal to 35 percent of calories.

Calories	Fat (g)	Calories	Fat (g)	Calories	Fat (g)
5	-----> 0.2	155	-----> 6.0	305	-----> 11.8
10	-----> 0.4	160	-----> 6.2	310	-----> 12.0
15	-----> 0.6	165	-----> 6.4	315	-----> 12.2
20	-----> 0.8	170	-----> 6.6	320	-----> 12.4
25	-----> 1.0	175	-----> 6.8	325	-----> 12.6
30	-----> 1.2	180	-----> 7.0	330	-----> 12.8
35	-----> 1.4	185	-----> 7.2	335	-----> 13.0
40	-----> 1.6	190	-----> 7.4	340	-----> 13.2
45	-----> 1.7	195	-----> 7.6	345	-----> 13.4
50	-----> 1.9	200	-----> 7.8	350	-----> 13.6
55	-----> 2.1	205	-----> 8.0	355	-----> 13.8
60	-----> 2.3	210	-----> 8.2	360	-----> 13.9
65	-----> 2.5	215	-----> 8.4	365	-----> 14.1
70	-----> 2.7	220	-----> 8.6	370	-----> 14.3
75	-----> 2.9	225	-----> 8.7	375	-----> 14.5
80	-----> 3.1	230	-----> 8.9	380	-----> 14.7
85	-----> 3.3	235	-----> 9.1	385	-----> 14.9
90	-----> 3.5	240	-----> 9.3	390	-----> 15.1
95	-----> 3.7	245	-----> 9.5	395	-----> 15.3
100	-----> 3.9	250	-----> 9.7	400	-----> 15.5
105	-----> 4.1	255	-----> 9.9	405	-----> 15.7
110	-----> 4.3	260	-----> 10.1	410	-----> 15.9
115	-----> 4.5	265	-----> 10.3	415	-----> 16.1
120	-----> 4.7	270	-----> 10.4	420	-----> 16.3
125	-----> 4.9	275	-----> 10.6	425	-----> 16.5
130	-----> 5.1	280	-----> 10.8	430	-----> 16.7
135	-----> 5.2	285	-----> 11.0	435	-----> 16.9
140	-----> 5.4	290	-----> 11.2	440	-----> 17.1
145	-----> 5.6	295	-----> 11.4	445	-----> 17.3
150	-----> 5.8	300	-----> 11.6	450	-----> 17.4

SHOPPERS' GUIDELINE -- 40% Fat

This table lists grams of fat which total 40 percent of calories. To use this table, look at a food label and find the number of calories per serving. Then find the corresponding number in the calories column of this guide which is closest to the number of calories on the product label. Now look to the next column in the same row, and you will find the number of grams of fat equal to 40 percent of calories.

Calories	Fat (g)	Calories	Fat (g)	Calories	Fat (g)
5	-----> 0.2	155	-----> 6.9	305	-----> 13.5
10	-----> 0.4	160	-----> 7.1	310	-----> 13.7
15	-----> 0.7	165	-----> 7.3	315	-----> 14.0
20	-----> 0.9	170	-----> 7.6	320	-----> 14.2
25	-----> 1.1	175	-----> 7.8	325	-----> 14.4
30	-----> 1.3	180	-----> 8.0	330	-----> 14.6
35	-----> 1.6	185	-----> 8.2	335	-----> 14.8
40	-----> 1.8	190	-----> 8.4	340	-----> 15.1
45	-----> 2.0	195	-----> 8.7	345	-----> 15.3
50	-----> 2.2	200	-----> 8.9	350	-----> 15.5
55	-----> 2.4	205	-----> 9.1	355	-----> 15.7
60	-----> 2.7	210	-----> 9.3	360	-----> 16.0
65	-----> 2.9	215	-----> 9.6	365	-----> 16.2
70	-----> 3.1	220	-----> 9.8	370	-----> 16.4
75	-----> 3.3	225	-----> 10.0	375	-----> 16.6
80	-----> 3.6	230	-----> 10.2	380	-----> 16.8
85	-----> 3.8	235	-----> 10.4	385	-----> 17.1
90	-----> 4.0	240	-----> 10.6	390	-----> 17.3
95	-----> 4.2	245	-----> 10.8	395	-----> 17.5
100	-----> 4.4	250	-----> 11.1	400	-----> 17.7
105	-----> 4.7	255	-----> 11.3	405	-----> 18.0
110	-----> 4.9	260	-----> 11.5	410	-----> 18.2
115	-----> 5.1	265	-----> 11.7	415	-----> 18.4
120	-----> 5.3	270	-----> 12.0	420	-----> 18.6
125	-----> 5.6	275	-----> 12.2	425	-----> 18.8
130	-----> 5.8	280	-----> 12.4	430	-----> 19.1
135	-----> 6.0	285	-----> 12.6	435	-----> 19.3
140	-----> 6.2	290	-----> 12.8	440	-----> 19.5
145	-----> 6.4	295	-----> 13.1	445	-----> 19.7
150	-----> 6.7	300	-----> 13.3	450	-----> 20.0

SHOPPERS' GUIDELINE -- 45% Fat

This table lists grams of fat which total 45 percent of calories. To use this table, look at a food label and find the number of calories per serving. Then find the corresponding number in the calories column of this guide which is closest to the number of calories on the product label. Now look to the next column in the same row, and you will find the number of grams of fat equal to 45 percent of calories.

Calories	Fat (g)	Calories	Fat (g)	Calories	Fat (g)
5	-----> 0.2	155	-----> 7.7	305	-----> 15.2
10	-----> 0.5	160	-----> 8.0	310	-----> 15.4
15	-----> 0.7	165	-----> 8.2	315	-----> 15.7
20	-----> 1.0	170	-----> 8.5	320	-----> 15.9
25	-----> 1.2	175	-----> 8.7	325	-----> 16.2
30	-----> 1.5	180	-----> 9.0	330	-----> 16.4
35	-----> 1.7	185	-----> 9.2	335	-----> 16.7
40	-----> 2.0	190	-----> 9.5	340	-----> 16.9
45	-----> 2.2	195	-----> 9.7	345	-----> 17.2
50	-----> 2.5	200	-----> 10.0	350	-----> 17.4
55	-----> 2.7	205	-----> 10.2	355	-----> 17.7
60	-----> 3.0	210	-----> 10.5	360	-----> 17.9
65	-----> 3.2	215	-----> 10.7	365	-----> 18.2
70	-----> 3.5	220	-----> 11.0	370	-----> 18.4
75	-----> 3.7	225	-----> 11.2	375	-----> 18.7
80	-----> 4.0	230	-----> 11.4	380	-----> 18.9
85	-----> 4.2	235	-----> 11.7	385	-----> 19.2
90	-----> 4.5	240	-----> 11.9	390	-----> 19.4
95	-----> 4.7	245	-----> 12.2	395	-----> 19.7
100	-----> 5.0	250	-----> 12.4	400	-----> 19.9
105	-----> 5.2	255	-----> 12.7	405	-----> 20.2
110	-----> 5.5	260	-----> 12.9	410	-----> 20.4
115	-----> 5.7	265	-----> 13.2	415	-----> 20.7
120	-----> 6.0	270	-----> 13.4	420	-----> 20.9
125	-----> 6.2	275	-----> 13.7	425	-----> 21.2
130	-----> 6.5	280	-----> 13.9	430	-----> 21.4
135	-----> 6.7	285	-----> 14.2	435	-----> 21.7
140	-----> 7.0	290	-----> 14.4	440	-----> 21.9
145	-----> 7.2	295	-----> 14.7	445	-----> 22.2
150	-----> 7.5	300	-----> 14.9	450	-----> 22.4

SHOPPERS' GUIDELINE -- 50% Fat

This table lists grams of fat which total 50 percent of calories. To use this table, look at a food label and find the number of calories per serving. Then find the corresponding number in the calories column of this guide which is closest to the number of calories on the product label. Now look to the next column in the same row, and you will find the number of grams of fat equal to 50 percent of calories.

Calories	Fat (g)	Calories	Fat (g)	Calories	Fat (g)
5	-----> 0.3	155	-----> 8.6	305	-----> 16.9
10	-----> 0.6	160	-----> 8.9	310	-----> 17.2
15	-----> 0.8	165	-----> 9.2	315	-----> 17.5
20	-----> 1.1	170	-----> 9.4	320	-----> 17.7
25	-----> 1.4	175	-----> 9.7	325	-----> 18.0
30	-----> 1.7	180	-----> 10.0	330	-----> 18.3
35	-----> 1.9	185	-----> 10.3	335	-----> 18.6
40	-----> 2.2	190	-----> 10.6	340	-----> 18.8
45	-----> 2.5	195	-----> 10.8	345	-----> 19.1
50	-----> 2.8	200	-----> 11.1	350	-----> 19.4
55	-----> 3.1	205	-----> 11.4	355	-----> 19.7
60	-----> 3.3	210	-----> 11.7	360	-----> 20.0
65	-----> 3.6	215	-----> 11.9	365	-----> 20.2
70	-----> 3.9	220	-----> 12.2	370	-----> 20.5
75	-----> 4.2	225	-----> 12.5	375	-----> 20.8
80	-----> 4.4	230	-----> 12.7	380	-----> 21.1
85	-----> 4.7	235	-----> 13.0	385	-----> 21.3
90	-----> 5.0	240	-----> 13.3	390	-----> 21.6
95	-----> 5.3	245	-----> 13.6	395	-----> 21.9
100	-----> 5.6	250	-----> 13.8	400	-----> 22.2
105	-----> 5.8	255	-----> 14.1	405	-----> 22.5
110	-----> 6.1	260	-----> 14.4	410	-----> 22.7
115	-----> 6.4	265	-----> 14.7	415	-----> 23.0
120	-----> 6.7	270	-----> 15.0	420	-----> 23.3
125	-----> 6.9	275	-----> 15.2	425	-----> 23.6
130	-----> 7.2	280	-----> 15.5	430	-----> 23.8
135	-----> 7.5	285	-----> 15.8	435	-----> 24.1
140	-----> 7.8	290	-----> 16.1	440	-----> 24.4
145	-----> 8.1	295	-----> 16.3	445	-----> 24.7
150	-----> 8.3	300	-----> 16.6	450	-----> 25.0

FOOD ANALYSIS

The following tool will enable you to determine the nutritional content of foods and identify low-calorie/low-fat substitute foods. In addition to aiding in the selection of foods, it will help you choose the best methods of preparation. Also, it will enable you to see the differences between types of fish or cuts of beef or poultry.

We have divided the foods into separate, logical categories (e.g., fruit and juice, dairy products, sandwiches, breakfast cereal, etc.), and within each category we use a uniform serving size. We have selected serving sizes for each category that represent a normal portion for most of the foods in the category. The uniform serving sizes within categories should simplify your food comparisons. To enable you to compare foods easily that are in different categories, we have selected serving sizes that are simple multiples of one another: 0.5, 1, 2, 4, and 8 ounces. Also, in the introduction to each of the 17 food categories, we list information on the average weight of specific foods (e.g., the average weight of an apple, a potato, a hot dog, etc.).

For almost every food, we have identified a substitute that is lower in calories and/or fat. For some healthful foods, the substitutes are not necessarily better foods, but are simply alternatives that are similarly low in fat and calories. In selecting these substitutes we attempted to choose foods that are reasonably similar in one way or another. To find a food that is even lower in calories and/or fat than the substitute, look up the substitute food, and you will see that it too has a substitute. For example, the substitute for "bacon, cured, cooked" is "Canadian bacon, cooked", and the substitute for "Canadian bacon, cooked" is "ham, canned, extra-lean", which in turn has as a substitute "turkey loaf breast".

The food analysis in this chapter is derived from U.S. Department of Agriculture information (*USDA Nutrient Database for Standard Reference* and *Nutritive Value of Foods*), supplemented by data from food companies. In this chapter we use the abbreviation "kcal" as the unit of measurement commonly called "Calories".

The following table is a list of the food categories and their corresponding serving sizes:

FOOD CATEGORY SERVING SIZES

No.	Food Category	Serving Size
1.	Beef, Pork and Lamb	8 ounces
2.	Beverages	8 ounces
3.	Bread, Bakery, Dessert & Candy	2 ounces
4.	Breakfast Cereal	1 ounce
5.	Chips, Crackers, Nuts & Seeds	1 ounce
6.	Dairy Products	4 ounces
7.	Fruit and Juice	4 ounces
8.	Miscellaneous Foods	4 ounces
9.	Pasta, Pizza and Rice	4 ounces
10.	Poultry	8 ounces
11.	Salad Dressings, Oils and Fats	0.5 ounce
12.	Sandwiches	4 ounces
13.	Sauces, Gravy and Condiments	0.5 ounce
14.	Seafood	8 ounces
15.	Soup	8 ounces
16.	Syrups, Jams and Preserves	0.5 ounce
17.	Vegetables and Salads	4 ounces

BEEF, PORK AND LAMB

Beef, pork and lamb are typically consumed as the main dish in a meal. Therefore, in order to facilitate comparison with other main-dish foods (i.e., chicken, seafood), we have selected a serving size of 8 ounces for this category. However, you should note that most foods in this category are relatively high in fat and therefore should be consumed in moderation. In order to stay within the Food and Nutrition Board recommendation of limiting fat intake to no more than 30% of total calories, you may need to consume smaller portions, perhaps 4 ounces rather than 8.

For your convenience, we have included some meat sandwiches and some foods made with beef (e.g., beef enchiladas, beef stew, beef potpie, etc.) in this category as well as in the Sandwiches category and the Miscellaneous Foods category respectively.

Weights and Measures

1. One medium-thickness slice of bacon cooked weighs approximately one-half ounce.
2. One hot dog weighs 1.6 ounces (for a package of 10 per pound).
3. One slice of lunch meat weighs approximately one ounce (e.g., one-pound package of bologna cut into 16 slices).

Serving size--8 ounces:	Calories kcal	Carbo grams	Prot grams	Fat grams	Fat % of kcal	Chol mg
Bacon, cured, cooked	1306	1.4	68.9	111.6	77	193
(canadian bacon, cooked)	420	2.9	54.9	19.1	41	132
Barbecue loaf, pork/beef	392	14.5	35.8	20.2	46	84
(turkey loaf breast)	249	0	51.0	3.6	13	93
Beef, arm, cooked	753	0	62.1	54.0	65	225
(beef, arm, lean, cooked)	490	0	74.8	18.8	35	229
Beef, arm, lean, cooked	490	0	74.8	18.8	35	229
(chicken breast, meat only, roasted)	374	0	70.3	8.2	20	193
Beef, chuck, pot roast, braised	693	0	63.9	48.0	63	227
(beef, chuck, pot roast, lean, braised)	480	0	74.6	18.6	36	227
Beef, chuck, pot roast, lean, braised	480	0	74.6	18.6	36	227
(chicken breast, meat only, roasted)	374	0	70.3	8.2	20	193

( ) indicates possible substitute foods that are lower in calories and/or fat.

Serving size--8 ounces:	Calories kcal	Carbo grams	Prot grams	Fat grams	Fat % of kcal	Chol mg
Beef, club steak, cooked	903	0	51.9	75.5	75	213
(beef, flank steak, lean, cooked)	469	0	61.5	22.9	44	152
Beef enchiladas	714	81.9	26.3	30.4	38	82
(bean burrito)	426	63.7	14.7	12.9	27	16
Beef, flank steak, cooked	513	0	59.9	28.3	50	154
(chicken breast, meat only, roasted)	374	0	70.3	8.2	20	193
Beef, flank steak, lean, cooked	469	0	61.5	22.9	44	152
(turkey, light, meat only, roasted)	356	0	67.8	7.3	18	156
Beef, hamburger, cooked	655	0	54.7	46.9	64	204
(turkey, fresh ground)	338	0	39.7	18.8	52	179
Beef, heart, cooked	397	0.9	65.3	12.7	29	438
(chicken breast, meat only, roasted)	374	0	70.3	8.2	20	193
Beef, hind shank, cooked	596	0	69.6	33.3	50	181
(beef, hind shank, lean, cooked)	456	0	76.4	14.5	29	177
Beef, hind shank, lean, cooked	456	0	76.4	14.5	29	177
(chicken breast, meat only, roasted)	374	0	70.3	8.2	20	193
Beef, hip-bone, sirloin, cooked	1000	0	47.6	88.5	80	213
(beef, sirloin steak, cooked)	610	0	62.6	37.9	56	204
Beef, kidneys, simmered	327	2.3	57.8	7.7	21	878
(beef, tripe, commercial)	227	0	43.3	4.5	18	154
Beef, liver, fried	492	17.7	60.6	18.1	33	1093
(chicken breast, meat only, roasted)	374	0	70.3	8.2	20	193
Beef, porterhouse, cooked	692	0	56.2	50.1	65	188
(beef, sirloin steak, cooked)	610	0	62.6	37.9	56	204
Beef potpie	435	40.8	16.6	22.5	47	41
(beef and vegetable stew, canned)	179	16.1	13.2	7.0	35	32
Beef, ribs (6th-12th), cooked	998	0	45.1	89.4	81	213
(beef, hind shank, lean, cooked)	456	0	76.4	14.5	29	177
Beef, round, cooked	544	0	61.9	30.8	51	181
(beef, hind shank, lean, cooked)	456	0	76.4	14.5	29	177
Beef, rump, cooked	787	0	53.5	61.9	71	213
(beef, rump, lean, cooked)	472	0	66.0	21.1	40	206
Beef, rump, lean, cooked	472	0	66.0	21.1	40	206
(beef, hind shank, lean, cooked)	456	0	76.4	14.5	29	177

( ) indicates possible substitute foods that are lower in calories and/or fat.

Serving size--8 ounces:	Calories kcal	Carbo grams	Prot grams	Fat grams	Fat % of kcal	Chol mg
Beef, short plate, cooked	980	0	50.6	84.6	78	213
(beef, hind shank, lean, cooked)	456	0	76.4	14.5	29	177
Beef, sirloin steak, cooked	610	0	62.6	37.9	56	204
(beef, flank steak, lean, cooked)	469	0	61.5	22.9	44	152
Beef stew	202	14.1	14.5	9.8	44	59
(beef chunky soup)	161	18.4	11.1	4.8	27	14
Beef, sweetbreads, cooked	726	0	58.7	52.6	65	1057
(chicken breast, meat only, roasted)	374	0	70.3	8.2	20	193
Beef, t-bone steak, cooked	676	0	56.7	48.1	64	188
(beef, sirloin steak, cooked)	610	0	62.6	37.9	56	204
Beef teriyaki	599	10.4	40.8	41.5	62	142
(beef, flank steak, lean, cooked)	469	0	61.5	22.9	44	152
Beef, tongue, medium fat, cooked	642	0.7	51.3	46.9	66	243
(chicken breast, meat only, roasted)	374	0	70.3	8.2	20	193
Beef, tongue, smoked	744	2.0	39.0	65.3	79	154
(chicken breast, meat only, roasted)	374	0	70.3	8.2	20	193
Beef, tripe, commercial	227	0	43.3	4.5	18	154
(beef, tripe, pickled)	141	0	26.8	2.9	19	154
Beef, tripe, pickled	141	0	26.8	2.9	19	154
(pickle, cucumber, dill)	24	5.0	1.6	0.4	15	0
Beerwurst, beef	746	3.9	28.1	67.8	82	138
(beerwurst, pork)	540	4.8	32.2	42.6	71	134
Beerwurst, pork	540	4.8	32.2	42.6	71	134
(turkey loaf breast)	249	0	51.0	3.6	13	93
Blood sausage	857	2.9	33.1	78.2	82	272
(sausage, new england brand)	365	10.9	39.2	17.2	42	111
Bologna, beef/pork	717	6.4	26.5	64.2	81	125
(turkey loaf breast)	249	0	51.0	3.6	13	93
Bratwurst, pork, cooked	683	4.8	32.0	58.7	77	136
(sausage, new england brand)	365	10.9	39.2	17.2	42	111
Braunschweiger, pork	814	7.0	30.6	72.8	80	354
(turkey loaf breast)	249	0	51.0	3.6	13	93
Canadian bacon, cooked	420	2.9	54.9	19.1	41	132
(ham, canned, extra-lean)	308	1.1	48.0	11.1	34	68

( ) indicates possible substitute foods that are lower in calories and/or fat.

Serving size--8 ounces:	Calories kcal	Carbo grams	Prot grams	Fat grams	Fat % of kcal	Chol mg
Cheese hot dog, pork/beef	742	3.4	31.8	65.5	79	154
(sausage, new england brand)	365	10.9	39.2	17.2	42	111
Cheeseburger sandwich	703	30.2	45.8	43.3	55	165
(grilled chicken sandwich)	474	40.1	53.1	9.8	19	133
Chili con carne with beans	302	27.7	17.0	13.8	41	39
(baked beans (without pork) canned)	272	52.2	14.3	1.1	4	0
Chili con carne without beans	454	13.2	23.4	33.6	67	59
(chili con carne with beans)	302	27.7	17.0	13.8	41	39
Chopped ham, canned	542	0.7	36.5	42.6	72	111
(ham, canned, extra-lean)	308	1.1	48.0	11.1	34	68
Corned beef, cooked	569	1.1	41.2	43.1	70	222
(corned beef, lean)	420	0	59.9	18.1	39	206
Corned beef hash	411	24.3	20.0	25.6	56	75
(ham, canned, extra-lean)	308	1.1	48.0	11.1	34	68
Corned beef, lean	420	0	59.9	18.1	39	206
(turkey loaf breast)	249	0	51.0	3.6	13	93
Dried chipped beef, cooked	349	16.1	18.6	23.4	60	91
(turkey loaf breast)	249	0	51.0	3.6	13	93
Dutch brand loaf, pork/beef	544	12.7	30.4	40.4	67	107
(turkey loaf breast)	249	0	51.0	3.6	13	93
Frankfurter (hot dog), beef/pork	726	5.7	25.6	66.0	82	113
(sausage, new england brand)	365	10.9	39.2	17.2	42	111
Ham and cheese loaf	587	3.2	37.6	45.8	70	129
(turkey loaf breast)	249	0	51.0	3.6	13	93
Ham and cheese spread	556	5.2	36.7	42.0	68	138
(turkey loaf breast)	249	0	51.0	3.6	13	93
Ham, canned	431	0	38.6	29.5	62	88
(ham, canned, extra-lean)	308	1.1	48.0	11.1	34	68
Ham, canned, extra-lean	308	1.1	48.0	11.1	34	68
(turkey loaf breast)	249	0	51.0	3.6	13	93
Ham croquette	569	26.5	37.0	34.2	54	159
(ham, canned, extra-lean)	308	1.1	48.0	11.1	34	68
Ham, cured, center	460	0	45.8	29.3	57	122
(ham, cured, extra-lean)	297	2.3	43.8	11.3	34	107

( ) indicates possible substitute foods that are lower in calories and/or fat.

Serving size--8 ounces:	Calories kcal	Carbo grams	Prot grams	Fat grams	Fat % of kcal	Chol mg
Ham, cured, extra-lean	297	2.3	43.8	11.3	34	107
(turkey loaf breast)	249	0	51.0	3.6	13	93
Ham, cured, lean	333	0	50.6	12.9	35	118
(ham, cured, extra-lean)	297	2.3	43.8	11.3	34	107
Ham, fresh, lean and fat, cooked	667	0	56.7	46.9	63	211
(ham, canned, extra-lean)	308	1.1	48.0	11.1	34	68
Ham, fresh, rump, lean, cooked	467	0	70	18.4	37	218
(ham, canned, extra-lean)	308	1.1	48.0	11.1	34	68
Ham, fresh, shank, cooked	655	0	57.3	45.6	64	208
(ham, canned, extra-lean)	308	1.1	48.0	11.1	34	68
Ham, fresh, shank, lean, cooked	488	0	64.0	23.8	44	209
(ham, canned, extra-lean)	308	1.1	48.0	11.1	34	68
Ham patties	714	3.9	29.0	64.0	81	159
(turkey loaf breast)	249	0	51.0	3.6	13	93
Ham salad spread	490	24.0	19.7	35.2	65	84
(turkey loaf breast)	249	0	51.0	3.6	13	93
Ham steak, extra-lean	277	0	44.5	9.8	32	102
(turkey loaf breast)	249	0	51.0	3.6	13	93
Hamburger on bun	691	76.8	31	29.7	38	88
(grilled chicken sandwich)	474	40.1	53.1	9.8	19	133
Hamburger on bun with cheese	703	30.2	45.8	43.3	55	165
(grilled chicken sandwich)	474	40.1	53.1	9.8	19	133
Hamburger w/bun, cheese, bacon	871	30.4	49.4	60.1	62	160
(grilled chicken sandwich)	474	40.1	53.1	9.8	19	133
Headcheese, pork	481	0.7	36.3	35.8	67	184
(sausage, new england brand)	365	10.9	39.2	17.2	42	111
Honey loaf, pork/beef	290	12.0	35.8	10.2	32	77
(turkey loaf breast)	249	0	51.0	3.6	13	93
Honey roll sausage, beef	413	5.0	42.2	23.8	52	113
(ham, canned, extra-lean)	308	1.1	48.0	11.1	34	68
Hot dog (frankfurter) on bun	560	41.7	24.0	33.5	53	102
(grilled chicken sandwich)	474	40.1	53.1	9.8	19	133
Italian sausage, pork, cooked	733	3.4	45.4	58.3	72	177
(sausage, new england brand)	365	10.9	39.2	17.2	42	111

( ) indicates possible substitute foods that are lower in calories and/or fat.

Serving size--8 ounces:	Calories kcal	Carbo grams	Prot grams	Fat grams	Fat % of kcal	Chol mg
Kielbasa, pork/beef	703	4.8	30.2	61.5	79	152
(turkey loaf breast)	249	0	51.0	3.6	13	93
Knockwurst, beef/pork	699	4.1	27.0	63.1	81	132
(chicken breast, meat only, roasted)	374	0	70.3	8.2	20	193
Lamb, heart, cooked	420	4.3	56.7	17.9	38	565
(beef, heart, cooked)	397	0.9	65.3	12.7	29	438
Lamb, leg, cooked	585	0	57.8	37.4	58	211
(lamb, leg, lean, cooked)	433	0	64.2	17.5	36	202
Lamb, leg, lean, cooked	433	0	64.2	17.5	36	202
(chicken breast, meat only, roasted)	374	0	70.3	8.2	20	193
Lamb, liver, broiled	499	5.7	69.4	20.0	36	1136
(lamb, leg, lean, cooked)	433	0	64.2	17.5	36	202
Lamb, loin, chop, broiled	717	0	57.2	52.4	66	227
(lamb, loin, lean, broiled)	490	0	68.0	22.0	40	215
Lamb, loin, lean, broiled	490	0	68.0	22.0	40	215
(chicken breast, meat only, roasted)	374	0	70.3	8.2	20	193
Lamb, rib, chops, broiled	819	0	50.1	67.1	74	225
(lamb, rib, lean, broiled)	533	0	62.8	29.3	49	206
Lamb, rib, lean, broiled	533	0	62.8	29.3	49	206
(chicken breast, meat only, roasted)	374	0	70.3	8.2	20	193
Lamb, shoulder, cooked	631	0	55.3	43.8	62	220
(lamb, shoulder, lean, cooked)	476	0	61.5	23.8	45	211
Lamb, shoulder, lean, cooked	476	0	61.5	23.8	45	211
(chicken breast, meat only, roasted)	374	0	70.3	8.2	20	193
Lamb, sweetbreads, cooked	397	0	63.7	13.8	31	1057
(chicken breast, meat only, roasted)	374	0	70.3	8.2	20	193
Lamb tongue, braised	624	0	49.0	46.0	66	429
(lamb, leg, lean, cooked)	433	0	64.2	17.5	36	202
Lebanon bologna, beef	513	6.1	43.7	29.9	57	159
(turkey loaf breast)	249	0	51.0	3.6	13	93
Liver cheese, pork	689	4.8	34.5	58.1	76	395
(chicken breast, meat only, roasted)	374	0	70.3	8.2	20	193
Liver pate	723	3.4	32.2	63.5	79	578
(chicken spread, canned)	435	12.2	34.9	26.5	55	118

( ) indicates possible substitute foods that are lower in calories and/or fat.

Serving size--8 ounces:	Calories kcal	Carbo grams	Prot grams	Fat grams	Fat % of kcal	Chol mg
Liverwurst, pork	739	5.0	32.0	64.6	79	358
(turkey loaf breast)	249	0	51.0	3.6	13	93
Luncheon sausage, pork/beef	590	3.6	34.9	47.4	72	145
(turkey loaf breast)	249	0	51.0	3.6	13	93
Lunchmeat, pork/beef	801	5.2	28.6	73.0	82	125
(turkey loaf breast)	249	0	51.0	3.6	13	93
Luxury loaf, pork	320	11.1	41.7	10.9	31	82
(turkey loaf breast)	249	0	51.0	3.6	13	93
Meatloaf	606	12.2	47.6	39.2	58	258
(turkey, light, meat only, roasted)	356	0	67.8	7.3	18	156
Olive loaf, pork	533	20.9	26.8	37.4	63	86
(turkey loaf breast)	249	0	51.0	3.6	13	93
Peppered loaf, pork/beef	336	10.4	39.2	14.5	39	104
(turkey loaf breast)	249	0	51.0	3.6	13	93
Pepperoni, pork/beef	1127	6.4	47.6	99.8	80	179
(turkey loaf breast)	249	0	51.0	3.6	13	93
Pickle pimento loaf, pork	594	13.4	26.1	47.9	73	84
(turkey loaf breast)	249	0	51.0	3.6	13	93
Picnic loaf, pork/beef	526	10.9	33.8	37.6	64	86
(turkey loaf breast)	249	0	51.0	3.6	13	93
Polish sausage, pork	739	3.6	32.0	65.1	79	159
(sausage, new england brand)	365	10.9	39.2	17.2	42	111
Pork blade, braised	732	0	49.6	57.6	72	193
(pork blade, lean, roasted)	560	0	60.3	33.5	56	211
Pork blade, broiled	725	0	51.0	56.2	71	195
(pork blade, lean, roasted)	560	0	60.3	33.5	56	211
Pork blade, fried	775	0	48.7	62.8	74	193
(pork blade, lean, roasted)	560	0	60.3	33.5	56	211
Pork blade, lean, braised	510	0	56.7	29.7	54	188
(pork tenderloin, lean, roasted)	372	0	63.7	10.9	28	179
Pork blade, lean, broiled	530	0	57.6	31.5	55	190
(pork tenderloin, lean, roasted)	372	0	63.7	10.9	28	179
Pork blade, lean, fried	546	0	56.0	34.2	58	186
(pork tenderloin, lean, roasted)	372	0	63.7	10.9	28	179

( ) indicates possible substitute foods that are lower in calories and/or fat.

Serving size--8 ounces:	Calories kcal	Carbo grams	Prot grams	Fat grams	Fat % of kcal	Chol mg
Pork blade, lean, roasted	560	0	60.3	33.5	56	211
(pork tenderloin, lean, roasted)	372	0	63.7	10.9	28	179
Pork blade, roasted	732	0	53.7	55.8	70	211
(pork blade, lean, roasted)	560	0	60.3	33.5	56	211
Pork brains, braised	313	0	27.4	21.5	62	5788
(beef, tripe, commercial)	227	0	43.3	4.5	18	154
Pork breakfast strip, cooked	1041	2.3	65.5	83.2	72	238
(canadian bacon, cooked)	420	2.9	54.9	19.1	41	132
Pork, brown and serve sausage	891	6.1	30.6	81.6	82	141
(sausage, new england brand)	365	10.9	39.2	17.2	42	111
Pork center rib, braised	567	0	60.5	34.2	56	165
(pork center rib, lean, roasted)	505	0	65.0	25.4	47	161
Pork center rib, broiled	778	0	55.8	59.9	69	211
(pork center rib, lean, roasted)	505	0	65.0	25.4	47	161
Pork center rib, fried	601	0	59.6	38.5	59	165
(pork center rib, lean, roasted)	505	0	65.0	25.4	47	161
Pork center rib, lean, braised	467	0	64.1	21.3	43	161
(pork tenderloin, lean, roasted)	372	0	63.7	10.9	28	179
Pork center rib, lean, broiled	496	0	69.8	22.0	41	184
(pork tenderloin, lean, roasted)	372	0	63.7	10.9	28	179
Pork center rib, lean, fried	494	0	63.7	24.7	47	159
(pork tenderloin, lean, roasted)	372	0	63.7	10.9	28	179
Pork center rib, lean, roasted	505	0	65.0	25.4	47	161
(pork tenderloin, lean, roasted)	372	0	63.7	10.9	28	179
Pork center rib, roasted	578	0	62.1	34.7	56	165
(pork center rib, lean, roasted)	505	0	65.0	25.4	47	161
Pork centerloin, braised	560	0	63.2	32.0	53	195
(pork centerloin, lean, broiled)	458	0	68.4	18.4	38	186
Pork centerloin, broiled	544	0	65.0	29.7	51	186
(pork centerloin, lean, broiled)	458	0	68.4	18.4	38	186
Pork centerloin, fried	628	0	67.8	37.6	56	208
(pork centerloin, lean, broiled)	458	0	68.4	18.4	38	186
Pork centerloin, lean, braised	458	0	67.5	18.8	39	193
(pork tenderloin, lean, roasted)	372	0	63.7	10.9	28	179

( ) indicates possible substitute foods that are lower in calories and/or fat.

Serving size--8 ounces:	Calories kcal	Carbo grams	Prot grams	Fat grams	Fat % of kcal	Chol mg
Pork centerloin, lean, broiled	458	0	68.4	18.4	38	186
(pork tenderloin, lean, roasted)	372	0	63.7	10.9	28	179
Pork centerloin, lean, fried	526	0	73	23.8	42	208
(pork tenderloin, lean, roasted)	372	0	63.7	10.9	28	179
Pork centerloin, lean, roasted	451	0	62.3	20.4	42	179
(pork tenderloin, lean, roasted)	372	0	63.7	10.9	28	179
Pork centerloin, roasted	530	0	59.6	30.6	54	181
(pork centerloin, lean, broiled)	458	0	68.4	18.4	38	186
Pork chitterlings, cooked	687	0	23.4	65.3	86	324
(ham, canned, extra-lean)	308	1.1	48.0	11.1	34	68
Pork, complete cuts, cooked	619	0	62.5	39	58	206
(pork, complete cuts, lean, cooked)	480	0	66.4	22	43	195
Pork, complete cuts, lean, cooked	480	0	66.4	22	43	195
(ham, canned, extra-lean)	308	1.1	48.0	11.1	34	68
Pork, country-style sausage	782	0	34.2	70.5	81	141
(sausage, new england brand)	365	10.9	39.2	17.2	42	111
Pork, deviled ham	796	0	31.5	73.3	83	147
(ham, canned, extra-lean)	308	1.1	48.0	11.1	34	68
Pork, feet, pickled	460	0	30.6	36.5	71	209
(ham, canned, extra-lean)	308	1.1	48.0	11.1	34	68
Pork, feet, simmered	440	0	43.5	28.1	57	227
(ham, canned, extra-lean)	308	1.1	48.0	11.1	34	68
Pork, fresh, spareribs, cooked	900	0	66.0	68.7	69	274
(pork tenderloin, lean, roasted)	372	0	63.7	10.9	28	179
Pork heart, braised	336	0.9	53.5	11.3	30	501
(ham, canned, extra-lean)	308	1.1	48.0	11.1	34	68
Pork, hog liver, fried	547	5.7	67.8	26.1	43	993
(pork tenderloin, lean, roasted)	372	0	63.7	10.9	28	179
Pork kidneys, braised	342	0	57.6	10.7	28	1089
(ham, canned, extra-lean)	308	1.1	48.0	11.1	34	68
Pork liver, braised	374	8.6	59.0	10.0	24	805
(ham, canned, extra-lean)	308	1.1	48.0	11.1	34	68
Pork loin (pork chops) braised	542	0	61.7	30.8	53	181
(pork loin, lean, roasted)	474	0	64.8	21.8	43	184

( ) indicates possible substitute foods that are lower in calories and/or fat.

Serving size--8 ounces:	Calories kcal	Carbo grams	Prot grams	Fat grams	Fat % of kcal	Chol mg
Pork loin (pork chops) broiled	548	0	61.9	31.5	53	181
(pork loin, lean, roasted)	474	0	64.8	21.8	43	184
Pork loin (pork chops) roasted	562	0	61.4	33.1	55	186
(pork tenderloin, lean, roasted)	372	0	63.7	10.9	28	179
Pork loin, lean, braised	462	0	64.8	20.6	42	179
(pork tenderloin, lean, roasted)	372	0	63.7	10.9	28	179
Pork loin, lean, broiled	476	0	64.8	22.2	44	179
(pork tenderloin, lean, roasted)	372	0	63.7	10.9	28	179
Pork loin, lean, roasted	474	0	64.8	21.8	43	184
(pork tenderloin, lean, roasted)	372	0	63.7	10.9	28	179
Pork lungs, braised	225	0	37.6	7.0	28	878
(beef, tripe, pickled)	141	0	26.8	2.9	19	154
Pork, sausage meat loaf	454	7.5	36.1	29.9	59	147
(chicken breast, meat only, roasted)	374	0	70.3	8.2	20	193
Pork, sausage meat, potted	562	0	39.7	43.5	70	177
(sausage, new england brand)	365	10.9	39.2	17.2	42	111
Pork, scrapple	488	33.1	20.0	30.8	57	100
(ham, canned, extra-lean)	308	1.1	48.0	11.1	34	68
Pork shoulder, cooked	662	0	52.8	48.5	67	204
(pork shoulder, lean, cooked)	521	0	57.3	30.6	55	204
Pork shoulder, lean, cooked	521	0	57.3	30.6	55	204
(pork tenderloin, lean, roasted)	372	0	63.7	10.9	28	179
Pork sirloin, braised	428	0	60.1	19.0	42	184
(pork tenderloin, lean, roasted)	372	0	63.7	10.9	28	179
Pork sirloin, broiled	471	0	69.1	19.5	39	206
(pork sirloin, lean, roasted)	449	0	65.3	18.8	39	195
Pork sirloin, lean, braised	397	0	61.2	15.0	36	184
(pork tenderloin, lean, roasted)	372	0	63.7	10.9	28	179
Pork sirloin, lean, broiled	437	0	70.5	15.2	33	208
(pork tenderloin, lean, roasted)	372	0	63.7	10.9	28	179
Pork sirloin, lean, roasted	449	0	65.3	18.8	39	195
(pork tenderloin, lean, roasted)	372	0	63.7	10.9	28	179
Pork sirloin, roasted	469	0	64.6	21.3	43	195
(pork sirloin, lean, roasted)	449	0	65.3	18.8	39	195

( ) indicates possible substitute foods that are lower in calories and/or fat.

Serving size--8 ounces:	Calories kcal	Carbo grams	Prot grams	Fat grams	Fat % of kcal	Chol mg
Pork, souse	411	2.7	29.5	30.4	67	147
(ham, canned, extra-lean)	308	1.1	48.0	11.1	34	68
Pork tenderloin, lean, roasted	372	0	63.7	10.9	28	179
(ham, canned, extra-lean)	308	1.1	48.0	11.1	34	68
Pork tongue, braised	615	0	54.7	42.2	62	331
(ham, canned, extra-lean)	308	1.1	48.0	11.1	34	68
Pork toploin, braised	528	0	62.8	28.8	51	170
(pork toploin, lean, roasted)	440	0	68.4	16.3	35	177
Pork toploin, broiled	519	0	68.0	25.4	46	184
(pork toploin, lean, roasted)	440	0	68.4	16.3	35	177
Pork toploin, fried	889	0	48.8	75.3	76	191
(pork toploin, lean, roasted)	440	0	68.4	16.3	35	177
Pork toploin, lean, braised	458	0	65.9	19.5	40	165
(pork tenderloin, lean, roasted)	372	0	63.7	10.9	28	179
Pork toploin, lean, broiled	460	0	70.5	17.7	36	181
(pork tenderloin, lean, roasted)	372	0	63.7	10.9	28	179
Pork toploin, lean, fried	583	0	63.5	34.7	54	184
(pork tenderloin, lean, roasted)	372	0	63.7	10.9	28	179
Pork toploin, lean, roasted	440	0	68.4	16.3	35	177
(pork tenderloin, lean, roasted)	372	0	63.7	10.9	28	179
Pork toploin, roasted	512	0	65.3	25.8	47	177
(pork toploin, lean, roasted)	440	0	68.4	16.3	35	177
Roast beef, canned	508	0	56.7	29.5	52	206
(turkey loaf breast)	249	0	51.0	3.6	13	93
Salami, beef/pork, cooked	567	5.2	31.5	45.6	72	147
(sausage, new england brand)	365	10.9	39.2	17.2	42	111
Sandwich spread, pork/beef	533	27.0	17.5	39.2	66	86
(turkey loaf breast)	249	0	51.0	3.6	13	93
Sausage, new england brand	365	10.9	39.2	17.2	42	111
(ham, canned, extra-lean)	308	1.1	48.0	11.1	34	68
Sausage, pork/beef, fresh, cooked	898	6.1	31.3	82.3	82	161
(sausage, new england brand)	365	10.9	39.2	17.2	42	111
Sausage, pork, fresh, cooked	837	2.3	44.5	70.8	76	188
(sausage, new england brand)	365	10.9	39.2	17.2	42	111

( ) indicates possible substitute foods that are lower in calories and/or fat.

Serving size--8 ounces:	Calories kcal	Carbo grams	Prot grams	Fat grams	Fat % of kcal	Chol mg
Sausage, smoked link, pork/beef	762	3.2	30.4	68.7	81	161
(sausage, new england brand)	365	10.9	39.2	17.2	42	111
Sausage, vienna, beef/pork	633	4.5	23.4	57.2	81	118
(sausage, new england brand)	365	10.9	39.2	17.2	42	111
Veal, chuck, medium fat, cooked	533	0	63.3	29.0	49	229
(chicken breast, meat only, roasted)	374	0	70.3	8.2	20	193
Veal, flank, cooked	885	0	52.6	73.3	75	229
(chicken breast, meat only, roasted)	374	0	70.3	8.2	20	193
Veal, fore shank, cooked	490	0	65.1	23.6	43	229
(chicken breast, meat only, roasted)	374	0	70.3	8.2	20	193
Veal parmesan	692	28.8	31.1	50.6	66	89
(chicken parmesan)	465	16.8	40.8	25.6	50	131
Veal scaloppine	592	10.7	49.9	36.3	55	208
(chicken breast, meat only, roasted)	374	0	70.3	8.2	20	193
Veal scaloppine (with cheese)	633	10.2	51.9	40.1	57	208
(chicken breast, meat only, roasted)	374	0	70.3	8.2	20	193

( ) indicates possible substitute foods that are lower in calories and/or fat.

BEVERAGES

Bevrg

The Beverage category includes everything from alcohol to water. For your convenience, we have included juices and dairy drinks in this category as well as in the Fruit and Juice category and Dairy category respectively. To facilitate comparisons, we have included information on powdered beverages (e.g., instant tea) in their prepared form only.

You will note that for alcoholic beverages the caloric content is not determined from carbohydrates, protein and fat alone; approximately 7 kcal are attributable to each gram of pure alcohol.

Weights and Measures

1. For beverages, one fluid ounce weighs approximately one ounce.
2. For beverages, one cup (8 fluid ounces) weighs approximately eight ounces (e.g., 1 cup milk weighs 8.6 ounces, 1 cup orange juice weighs 8.7 ounces, 1 cup coffee weighs 8.5 ounces, 1 cup 100 proof alcohol weighs 7.9 ounces).

Serving size--8 ounces:	Calories kcal	Carbo grams	Prot grams	Fat grams	Fat % of kcal	Chol mg
Alcohol: 100-proof gin, rum, etc.	669	0	0	0	0	0
(club soda)	0	0	0	0	0	0
Alcohol: 90-proof gin, rum, etc.	596	0	0	0	0	0
(club soda)	0	0	0	0	0	0
Alcohol: 86-proof gin, rum, etc.	565	0	0	0	0	0
(club soda)	0	0	0	0	0	0
Alcohol: 80-proof gin, rum, etc.	524	0	0	0	0	0
(club soda)	0	0	0	0	0	0
Apple cider	95	23.4	0.2	0.2	2	0
(tomato juice)	39	9.5	1.8	0.2	5	0
Apple juice	95	23.4	0.2	0.2	2	0
(tomato juice)	39	9.5	1.8	0.2	5	0
Apricot nectar	127	32.7	0.9	0.2	1	0
(orange juice, fresh)	102	23.6	1.6	0.5	4	0
Beef broth and tomato juice	84	19.3	1.4	0.2	2	0
(tomato juice)	39	9.5	1.8	0.2	5	0

( ) indicates possible substitute foods that are lower in calories and/or fat.

Serving size--8 ounces:	Calories kcal	Carbo grams	Prot grams	Fat grams	Fat % of kcal	Chol mg
Beer	95	8.6	0.7	0	0	0
(light beer: miller lite)	64	1.8	0.7	0	0	0
Blackberry juice	84	17.7	0.7	1.4	15	0
(tomato juice)	39	9.5	1.8	0.2	5	0
Bloody mary	177	7.5	1.1	0.2	1	0
(tomato juice)	39	9.5	1.8	0.2	5	0
Bourbon and soda	204	0	0	0	0	0
(club soda)	0	0	0	0	0	0
Buttermilk	91	10.9	7.5	2.0	20	8
(milk, skim)	79	10.9	7.7	0.5	6	4
Carrot juice	91	21.1	2.0	0.2	2	0
(tomato juice)	39	9.5	1.8	0.2	5	0
Cereal beverage (with milk)	147	12.7	7.5	7.5	46	0
(cereal beverage (with water))	11	2.3	0.2	0	0	0
Cereal beverage (with water)	11	2.3	0.2	0	0	0
(coffee, black)	2	0	0	0	0	0
Chocolate milk, 1% low fat	143	23.6	7.3	2.3	14	7
(milk, skim)	79	10.9	7.7	0.5	6	4
Chocolate milk, 2% low fat	163	23.6	7.3	4.5	25	15
(chocolate milk, 1% low fat)	143	23.6	7.3	2.3	14	7
Chocolate milk, whole	188	23.4	7.3	7.7	37	28
(chocolate milk, 1% low fat)	143	23.6	7.3	2.3	14	7
Clam and tomato juice	104	24.7	1.4	0.2	2	0
(tomato juice)	39	9.5	1.8	0.2	5	0
Club soda	0	0	0	0	0	0
(no alternate identified)						
Coconut milk	522	12.5	5.2	54.0	93	0
(pineapple juice)	127	31.3	0.7	0.2	1	0
Coffee, black	2	0	0	0	0	0
(water)	0	0	0	0	0	0
Coffee liqueur	762	106.1	0.2	0.7	1	0
(coffee, black)	2	0	0	0	0	0
Coffee with cream	48	0.9	0.7	4.3	81	15
(coffee, black)	2	0	0	0	0	0

( ) indicates possible substitute foods that are lower in calories and/or fat.

Serving size--8 ounces:	Calories kcal	Carbo grams	Prot grams	Fat grams	Fat % of kcal	Chol mg
Coffee with cream and sugar	91	12.2	0.7	4.3	43	15
(coffee, black)	2	0	0	0	0	0
Cola: coke, pepsi, rc, etc	88	22.7	0	0	0	0
(diet soda: diet coke, diet pepsi)	0	0	0	0	0	0
Cranberry-apple juice drink	152	38.8	0.2	0	0	0
(cranberry cocktail, low calorie)	43	10.7	0	0	0	0
Cranberry-apricot juice drink	145	36.7	0.5	0	0	0
(cranberry cocktail, low calorie)	43	10.7	0	0	0	0
Cranberry-grape juice drink	127	31.8	0.5	0.2	1	0
(cranberry cocktail, low calorie)	43	10.7	0	0	0	0
Cranberry cocktail, low calorie	43	10.7	0	0	0	0
(diet soda: diet coke, diet pepsi)	2	0.2	0.2	0	0	0
Cranberry juice cocktail	132	33.8	0	0	0	0
(cranberry cocktail, low calorie)	43	10.7	0	0	0	0
Cream soda	116	30.1	0	0	0	0
(diet soda: diet coke, diet pepsi)	2	0.2	0.2	0	0	0
Creme de menthe	841	94.3	0	0.7	1	0
(diet soda: diet coke, diet pepsi)	2	0.2	0.2	0	0	0
Daiquiri	422	15.4	0.2	0.2	0	0
(pineapple juice, canned)	127	31.3	0.7	0.2	1	0
Diet soda: diet coke, diet pepsi	2	0.2	0.2	0	0	0
(Club soda)	0	0	0	0	0	0
Eggnog	306	30.6	8.6	17.0	50	133
(chocolate milk, 1% low fat)	143	23.6	7.3	2.3	14	7
Fruit punch drink	107	27.0	0	0	0	0
(diet soda: diet coke, diet pepsi)	2	0.2	0.2	0	0	0
Gin and tonic	172	15.9	0	0	0	0
(club soda)	0	0	0	0	0	0
Ginger ale	70	18.1	0	0	0	0
(diet soda: diet coke, diet pepsi)	2	0.2	0.2	0	0	0
Grape drink	102	26.1	0	0	0	0
(diet soda: diet coke, diet pepsi)	2	0.2	0.2	0	0	0
Grape juice	138	34.0	1.4	0.2	1	0
(orange juice, fresh)	102	23.6	1.6	0.5	4	0

( ) indicates possible substitute foods that are lower in calories and/or fat.

Serving size--8 ounces:	Calories kcal	Carbo grams	Prot grams	Fat grams	Fat % of kcal	Chol mg
Grape soda	98	25.4	0	0	0	0
(diet soda: diet coke, diet pepsi)	2	0.2	0.2	0	0	0
Grapefruit drink, canned	122	31.3	0.2	0	0	0
(grapefruit juice, fresh-squeezed)	88	20.9	1.1	0.2	2	0
Grapefruit juice, canned, sweetened	104	25.2	1.4	0.2	2	0
(grapefruit juice, fresh-squeezed)	88	20.9	1.1	0.2	2	0
Grapefruit juice, fresh-squeezed	88	20.9	1.1	0.2	2	0
(tomato juice)	39	9.5	1.8	0.2	5	0
Hot cocoa	197	23.4	8.2	8.2	37	30
(chocolate milk, 1% low fat)	143	23.6	7.3	2.3	14	7
Imitation milk with vegetable oil	138	14.1	4.1	7.7	50	0
(milk, skim)	79	10.9	7.7	0.5	6	4
Kahlua	762	106.1	0.2	0.7	1	0
(coffee, black)	2	0	0	0	0	0
Lemon-lime soda (7up, sprite)	91	23.6	0	0	0	0
(diet soda: diet coke, diet pepsi)	2	0.2	0.2	0	0	0
Lemon juice, fresh	57	19.5	0.9	0	0	0
(chili sauce, hot, green)	45	11.3	1.6	0.2	4	0
Lemonade	91	23.8	0.2	0	0	0
(diet soda: diet coke, diet pepsi)	2	0.2	0.2	0	0	0
Light beer: amstel light	64	3.4	0.7	0	0	0
(diet soda: diet coke, diet pepsi)	2	0.2	0.2	0	0	0
Light beer: blatz light	64	2.0	0.7	0	0	0
(diet soda: diet coke, diet pepsi)	2	0.2	0.2	0	0	0
Light beer: bud light	88	8.2	0.7	0	0	0
(diet soda: diet coke, diet pepsi)	2	0.2	0.2	0	0	0
Light beer: coors light	70	3.4	0.5	0	0	0
(diet soda: diet coke, diet pepsi)	2	0.2	0.2	0	0	0
Light beer: labatt's light	77	5.9	0.7	0	0	0
(diet soda: diet coke, diet pepsi)	2	0.2	0.2	0	0	0
Light beer: michelob light	88	8.2	0.7	0	0	0
(diet soda: diet coke, diet pepsi)	2	0.2	0.2	0	0	0
Light beer: miller lite	64	1.8	0.7	0	0	0
(diet soda: diet coke, diet pepsi)	2	0.2	0.2	0	0	0

( ) indicates possible substitute foods that are lower in calories and/or fat.

Serving size--8 ounces:	Calories kcal	Carbo grams	Prot grams	Fat grams	Fat % of kcal	Chol mg
Light beer: natural light	73	4.3	0.9	0	0	0
(diet soda: diet coke, diet pepsi)	2	0.2	0.2	0	0	0
Light beer: old milwaukee light	79	6.1	0.5	0	0	0
(diet soda: diet coke, diet pepsi)	2	0.2	0.2	0	0	0
Light beer: schaefer light	75	5.9	0.5	0	0	0
(diet soda: diet coke, diet pepsi)	2	0.2	0.2	0	0	0
Lime juice, fresh	61	20.4	0.9	0.2	3	0
(lemon juice, fresh)	57	19.5	0.9	0	0	0
Limeade	93	24.9	0	0	0	0
(diet soda: diet coke, diet pepsi)	2	0.2	0.2	0	0	0
Manhattan	508	7.3	0.2	0	0	0
(club soda)	0	0	0	0	0	0
Martini	506	0.7	0	0	0	0
(club soda)	0	0	0	0	0	0
Milk, 1% low fat	95	10.9	7.5	2.5	24	9
(milk, skim)	79	10.9	7.7	0.5	6	4
Milk, 2% low fat	113	10.9	7.5	4.3	34	17
(milk, skim)	79	10.9	7.7	0.5	6	4
Milk, goat, whole	156	10.0	8.2	9.3	54	26
(milk, skim)	79	10.9	7.7	0.5	6	4
Milk shake, chocolate	288	46.5	7.7	8.4	26	29
(chocolate milk, 1% low fat)	143	23.6	7.3	2.3	14	7
Milk shake, strawberry	256	42.9	7.7	6.4	23	0
(chocolate milk, 1% low fat)	143	23.6	7.3	2.3	14	7
Milk shake, vanilla	254	40.4	8.8	6.8	24	27
(milk, 1% low fat)	95	10.9	7.5	2.5	24	9
Milk, sheep, whole	245	12.2	13.6	15.9	58	61
(milk, skim)	79	10.9	7.7	0.5	6	4
Milk, skim	79	10.9	7.7	0.5	6	4
(water)	0	0	0	0	0	0
Milk, whole, 3.3% fat	138	10.7	7.5	7.5	49	31
(milk, skim)	79	10.9	7.7	0.5	6	4
Milk, whole, 3.7% fat	145	10.4	7.5	8.4	52	32
(milk, skim)	79	10.9	7.7	0.5	6	4

( ) indicates possible substitute foods that are lower in calories and/or fat.

Serving size--8 ounces:	Calories kcal	Carbo grams	Prot grams	Fat grams	Fat % of kcal	Chol mg
Orange-apricot juice drink	113	28.8	0.7	0.2	2	0
(orange juice, fresh)	102	23.6	1.6	0.5	4	0
Orange breakfast drink, prepared	104	26.8	0	0	0	0
(orange juice, fresh)	102	23.6	1.6	0.5	4	0
Orange juice, fresh	102	23.6	1.6	0.5	4	0
(tomato juice)	39	9.5	1.8	0.2	5	0
Orange soda	109	27.9	0	0	0	0
(diet soda: diet coke, diet pepsi)	2	0.2	0.2	0	0	0
Papaya nectar	129	32.9	0.5	0.2	1	0
(orange juice, fresh)	102	23.6	1.6	0.5	4	0
Pear nectar	136	35.8	0.2	0	0	0
(orange juice, fresh)	102	23.6	1.6	0.5	4	0
Pina colada	422	64.2	0.9	4.3	9	0
(pineapple juice, canned)	127	31.3	0.7	0.2	1	0
Pineapple-orange juice drink	113	26.7	2.9	0	0	0
(orange juice, fresh)	102	23.6	1.6	0.5	4	0
Pineapple juice	127	31.3	0.7	0.2	1	0
(orange juice, fresh)	102	23.6	1.6	0.5	4	0
Prune juice	161	39.5	1.4	0	0	0
(orange juice, fresh)	102	23.6	1.6	0.5	4	0
Quinine water	70	18.1	0	0	0	0
(club soda)	0	0	0	0	0	0
Root beer	93	23.8	0	0	0	0
(diet soda: diet coke, diet pepsi)	2	0.2	0.2	0	0	0
Screwdriver	186	19.5	1.1	0	0	0
(orange juice, fresh)	102	23.6	1.6	0.5	4	0
Tangerine juice	98	22.9	1.1	0.5	5	0
(tomato juice)	39	9.5	1.8	0.2	5	0
Tangelo juice	93	22.0	1.1	0.2	2	0
(tomato juice)	39	9.5	1.8	0.2	5	0
Tea, brewed	2	0.7	0	0	0	0
(water)	0	0	0	0	0	0
Tea, instant w/sugar, prepared	77	19.3	0.2	0	0	0
(tea, low-cal instant, prepared)	5	1.1	0	0	0	0

( ) indicates possible substitute foods that are lower in calories and/or fat.

Bevrg

Serving size--8 ounces:	Calories kcal	Carbo grams	Prot grams	Fat grams	Fat % of kcal	Chol mg
Tea, low-cal instant, prepared	2	0.5	0	0	0	0
(water)	0	0	0	0	0	0
Tequila sunrise	249	19.5	0.7	0.2	1	0
(orange juice, fresh)	102	23.6	1.6	0.5	4	0
Tom collins	125	2.9	0	0	0	0
(club soda)	0	0	0	0	0	0
Tomato juice	39	9.5	1.8	0.2	5	0
(club soda)	0	0	0	0	0	0
Tonic water	77	20.0	0	0	0	0
(club soda)	0	0	0	0	0	0
Vegetable juice cocktail	43	10.2	1.4	0.2	4	0
(tomato juice)	39	9.5	1.8	0.2	5	0
Vodka martini	506	0.7	0	0	0	0
(club soda)	0	0	0	0	0	0
Water	0	0	0	0	0	0
(no alternate identified)						
Whiskey sour	308	12.7	0.5	0.2	1	0
(club soda)	0	0	0	0	0	0
Wine, dessert	311	17.5	0.2	0	0	0
(wine, white)	154	1.8	0.2	0	0	0
Wine, red	163	3.9	0.5	0	0	0
(grape juice)	138	34.0	1.4	0.2	1	0
Wine, rose	161	3.2	0.5	0	0	0
(grape juice)	138	34.0	1.4	0.2	1	0
Wine, white	154	1.8	0.2	0	0	0
(grape juice)	138	34.0	1.4	0.2	1	0

( ) indicates possible substitute foods that are lower in calories and/or fat.

BREAD, BAKERY, DESSERT & CANDY

The foods in this category are displayed with a serving size of 2 ounces. The normal serving sizes for items in this category vary greatly because of the broad range of different types of food products. We selected 2 ounces because it seemed like a reasonable middle ground between the small/light-weight serving items (e.g., hard candies, gum drops, etc.) and the large/heavy-weight serving items (e.g., ice cream, pies, etc.). Also, the arithmetic to convert from 2 ounces to either 1 ounce or 4 ounces is simple.

Weights and Measures

1. One slice of bread weighs approximately 1 ounce.
2. One piece of pie (1/8 of a 9" diameter pie) weighs approximately four ounces.
3. One cupcake (2.5" to 2.75" diameter) weighs approximately one ounce.
4. One bagel weighs approximately two ounces.
5. One fig bar (1.5" x 1.75" x 0.5") weighs approximately one-half ounce.
6. Four cookies (2" diameter, 1/4" thick) weigh approximately one ounce.
7. One doughnut (cake type 3 5/8" diameter, 1 1/4" high) weighs approximately two ounces.
8. Ten jellybeans (3/4" long, 1/2" wide) weigh approximately one ounce.
9. Four marshmallows weigh approximately one ounce.
10. One cup ice cream weighs approximately five ounces.

Serving size--2 ounces:	Calories kcal	Carbo grams	Prot grams	Fat grams	Fat % of kcal	Chol mg
Angel food cake	153	34.1	4.0	0.1	1	0
(bread, boston brown)	120	25.9	3.1	0.7	5	1
Apple brown betty	86	16.8	0.9	2.0	21	5
(applesauce, canned, unsweetened)	24	6.4	0.1	0	0	0
Apple pie	150	21.0	1.4	7.1	42	0
(apple brown betty)	86	16.8	0.9	2.0	21	5

( ) indicates possible substitute foods that are lower in calories and/or fat.

Serving size--2 ounces:	Calories kcal	Carbo grams	Prot grams	Fat grams	Fat % of kcal	Chol mg
Apricots, candied	192	49.0	0.3	0.1	0	0
(apricots, fresh)	27	6.3	0.8	0.2	7	0
Bagel, egg	158	30.0	6.0	1.2	7	14
(english muffin, plain)	133	26.1	4.4	1.0	7	0
Bagel, onion	162	31.4	7.1	1.0	6	0
(english muffin, plain)	133	26.1	4.4	1.0	7	0
Bagel, plain	156	30.3	5.9	0.9	5	0
(english muffin, plain)	133	26.1	4.4	1.0	7	0
Bagel, raisin & honey w/cinnamon	160	32.0	6.4	0.8	4	0
(english muffin, plain)	133	26.1	4.4	1	7	0
Bagel, rye/pumpernickel	152	30.4	6.1	1.0	6	0
(english muffin, plain)	133	26.1	4.4	1.0	7	0
Bagel, whole wheat	151	30.1	6.2	1.1	7	0
(english muffin, plain)	133	26.1	4.4	1.0	7	0
Bagel with cream cheese	166	21.7	5.6	6.7	36	19
(bagel, plain)	156	30.3	5.9	0.9	5	0
Banana custard pie	125	17.4	2.6	5.3	38	36
(low-calorie pudding, prepared)	32	5.6	1.9	0	0	0
Biscuits	201	25.3	4.0	9.2	41	2
(english muffin, plain)	133	26.1	4.4	1.0	7	0
Bitter chocolate	296	16.0	5.8	31.3	76	0
(candy, chocolate fudge)	216	45.0	1.0	4.8	19	8
Blackberry pie	138	19.5	1.5	6.2	40	0
(blackberries, fresh)	29	7.3	0.4	0.2	6	0
Blueberry pie	137	19.8	1.4	6.1	40	6
(blueberries, fresh)	32	8.0	0.4	0.2	6	0
Bread, american rye	148	27.4	4.8	1.9	12	0
(low-calorie rye bread)	108	24.3	5.4	0.7	6	0
Bread, boston brown	120	25.9	3.1	0.7	5	1
(low-calorie wheat bread)	100	15.0	5.0	2.1	19	0
Bread, french	155	29.4	5.0	1.7	10	0
(low-calorie white bread)	100	17.5	5.0	2.1	19	0
Bread, italian	154	28.3	5.0	2.0	12	0
(low-calorie white bread)	100	17.5	5.0	2.1	19	0

( ) indicates possible substitute foods that are lower in calories and/or fat.

Serving size--2 ounces:	Calories kcal	Carbo grams	Prot grams	Fat grams	Fat % of kcal	Chol mg
Bread pudding/raisin	106	16.1	3.2	3.5	30	39
(low-calorie pudding, prepared)	32	5.6	1.9	0	0	0
Bread, pumpernickel rye	142	26.9	4.9	1.8	11	0
(low-calorie rye bread)	108	24.3	5.4	0.7	6	0
Bread, raisin	155	29.6	4.5	2.5	14	0
(bread, boston brown)	120	25.9	3.1	0.7	5	1
Bread stuffing mix, cooked	101	12.3	1.8	4.9	44	0
(potatoes, baked, without skin)	53	12.2	1.1	0.1	2	0
Bread, white	147	26.7	5.2	2.3	14	0
(low-calorie white bread)	100	17.5	5.0	2.1	19	0
Bread, whole wheat	139	26.1	5.5	2.4	15	0
(low-calorie wheat bread)	100	15.0	5.0	2.1	19	0
Brown and serve rolls	170	28.7	4.5	3.9	21	4
(bread, boston brown)	120	25.9	3.1	0.7	5	1
Brownies	230	36.8	3.1	9.5	37	9
(angel food cake)	153	34.1	4.0	0.1	1	0
Brownies with nuts	275	28.9	3.7	17.7	58	47
(angel food cake)	153	34.1	4.0	0.1	1	0
Butterscotch pie	158	18.9	2.7	8.1	46	35
(low-calorie pudding, prepared)	32	5.6	1.9	0	0	0
Cake, boston cream pie	178	26.2	2.6	7.5	37	26
(low-calorie pudding, prepared)	32	5.6	1.9	0	0	0
Cake, cottage pudding	159	27.2	2.9	4.6	26	36
(low-calorie pudding, prepared)	32	5.6	1.9	0	0	0
Cake, gingerbread	202	27.9	2.2	9.3	41	18
(angel food cake)	153	34.1	4.0	0.1	1	0
Cake icing, caramel	204	43.4	0.7	3.8	17	12
(chocolate syrup, thin type)	139	35.6	1.3	1.1	7	0
Cake icing, chocolate	225	35.8	0.6	10	38	0
(chocolate syrup, thin type)	139	35.6	1.3	1.1	7	0
Cake icing, chocolate fudge	214	38.0	1.2	8.2	34	11
(chocolate syrup, thin type)	139	35.6	1.3	1.1	7	0
Cake icing, coconut	233	29.9	0.8	13.6	50	0
(chocolate syrup, thin type)	139	35.6	1.3	1.1	7	0

( ) indicates possible substitute foods that are lower in calories and/or fat.

Serving size--2 ounces:	Calories kcal	Carbo grams	Prot grams	Fat grams	Fat % of kcal	Chol mg
Cake icing, cream fudge	217	37.4	1.5	8.6	36	0
(chocolate syrup, thin type)	139	35.6	1.3	1.1	7	0
Cake icing, white	138	35.5	0.8	0	0	0
(dessert topping, ready to eat)	107	9.4	2.0	7.0	59	6
Candied figs	170	41.8	2.0	0.1	1	0
(figs, fresh)	42	10.9	0.5	0.2	4	0
Candied grapefruit peel	179	45.7	0.2	0.2	1	0
(grapefruit, fresh)	18	4.6	0.3	0.1	5	0
Candied lemon peel	179	45.7	0.2	0.2	1	0
(lemon without peel)	16	5.3	0.6	0.2	11	0
Candied orange peel	179	45.7	0.2	0.2	1	0
(orange, fresh)	27	6.7	0.5	0.1	2	0
Candied pineapple	179	45.4	0.5	0.2	1	0
(pineapple, fresh)	28	7.0	0.2	0.2	6	0
Candy, bittersweet chocolate	270	26.5	4.5	22.5	75	0
(candy, chocolate-flavored caramel)	204	49.5	1.1	1.4	6	0
Candy, butterscotch	225	53.8	0	1.9	8	6
(hard candy)	211	55.6	0	0	0	0
Candy, caramels	216	43.6	2.6	4.6	18	4
(hard candy)	211	55.6	0	0	0	0
Candy, caramels with nuts	243	40.0	2.6	9.2	34	1
(candy, caramels)	216	43.6	2.6	4.6	18	4
Candy, chocolate-flavored caramel	204	49.5	1.1	1.4	6	0
(candy, marshmallows)	180	46.1	1.0	0.1	0	0
Candy, chocolate fudge	216	45.0	1.0	4.8	19	8
(hard candy)	211	55.6	0	0	0	0
Candy, chocolate fudge with nuts	241	41.2	1.9	9.1	32	8
(candy, chocolate fudge)	216	45.0	1.0	4.8	19	8
Candy, fondant	203	52.6	0	0	0	0
(candy, marshmallows)	180	46.1	1.0	0.1	0	0
Candy, gum drops	219	56.0	0	0	0	0
(candy, marshmallows)	180	46.1	1.0	0.1	0	0
Candy, jelly beans	208	52.8	0	0.3	1	0
(candy, marshmallows)	180	46.1	1.0	0.1	0	0

( ) indicates possible substitute foods that are lower in calories and/or fat.

Serving size--2 ounces:	Calories kcal	Carbo grams	Prot grams	Fat grams	Fat % of kcal	Chol mg
Candy, marshmallows	180	46.1	1.0	0.1	0	0
(angel food cake)	153	34.1	4.0	0.1	1	0
Candy, milk chocolate with almonds	302	29.1	5.3	20.2	60	10
(candy, peanut brittle)	257	39.3	4.2	10.8	36	7
Candy, milk chocolate with peanuts	308	25.3	8.0	21.6	63	7
(candy, peanut brittle)	257	39.3	4.2	10.8	36	7
Candy, peanut bars	296	26.9	8.8	19.1	55	4
(candy, peanut brittle)	257	39.3	4.2	10.8	36	7
Candy, peanut brittle	257	39.3	4.2	10.8	36	7
(candy, gum drops)	219	56	0	0	0	0
Candy, plain milk chocolate	291	33.6	3.9	17.3	51	12
(candy, chocolate-flavored caramel)	204	49.5	1.1	1.4	6	0
Candy, sweet chocolate	286	33.8	2.2	19.4	55	0
(candy, chocolate-flavored caramel)	204	49.5	1.1	1.4	6	0
Candy, vanilla fudge	209	46.6	0.6	3.1	13	9
(candy, marshmallows)	180	46.1	1.0	0.1	0	0
Candy, vanilla fudge with nuts	235	42.6	1.6	7.5	28	8
(candy, vanilla fudge)	209	46.6	0.6	3.1	13	9
Cane syrup	149	38.6	0	0	0	0
(low-calorie syrup)	44	11.9	0	0	0	0
Caramel cake, no icing	218	30.4	2.6	9.8	40	44
(angel food cake)	153	34.1	4.0	0.1	1	0
Caramel cake with icing	205	32.6	2.1	7.7	34	53
(angel food cake)	153	34.1	4.0	0.1	1	0
Carrot cake	194	26.5	2.9	8.9	41	41
(angel food cake)	153	34.1	4.0	0.1	1	0
Charlotte russe	162	19.0	3.3	8.3	46	112
(low-calorie pudding, prepared)	32	5.6	1.9	0	0	0
Cheese souffle	124	3.5	5.6	9.7	70	105
(low-calorie pudding, prepared)	32	5.6	1.9	0	0	0
Cheesecake	182	14.4	3.1	12.7	62	31
(angel food cake)	153	34.1	4.0	0.1	1	0
Cherry pie	153	21.8	1.5	6.9	40	6
(cherries, sweet, fresh)	41	9.4	0.7	0.6	13	0

( ) indicates possible substitute foods that are lower in calories and/or fat.

Serving size--2 ounces:	Calories kcal	Carbo grams	Prot grams	Fat grams	Fat % of kcal	Chol mg
Chocolate cake, no icing	173	27.8	3.2	6.6	32	31
(angel food cake)	153	34.1	4.0	0.1	1	0
Chocolate cake w/chocolate icing	208	30.9	2.3	9.3	39	26
(angel food cake)	153	34.1	4.0	0.1	1	0
Chocolate cake with white icing	209	33.6	2.2	8.3	36	27
(angel food cake)	153	34.1	4.0	0.1	1	0
Chocolate chiffon pie	186	24.8	3.9	8.7	42	75
(chocolate meringue pie)	143	19.0	2.7	6.8	43	35
Chocolate-coated almonds	323	22.5	7.0	24.8	69	1
(sugar-coated almonds)	259	39.8	4.4	10.5	36	0
Chocolate-coated chocolate fudge	244	41.4	2.2	9.1	34	1
(candy, chocolate-flavored caramel)	204	49.5	1.1	1.4	6	0
Chocolate-coated coconut	248	40.8	1.6	10.0	36	1
(chocolate-coated fondant)	232	45.9	1.0	6.0	23	1
Chocolate-coated fondant	232	45.9	1.0	6.0	23	1
(candy, chocolate-flavored caramel)	204	49.5	1.1	1.4	6	0
Chocolate-coated fudge with nuts	256	38.2	2.8	11.8	41	1
(candy, chocolate-flavored caramel)	204	49.5	1.1	1.4	6	0
Chocolate-coated hard candy	263	40.0	3.7	11.1	38	1
(hard candy)	211	55.6	0	0	0	0
Chocolate-coated nougat & caramel	236	41.3	2.3	7.9	30	3
(candy, chocolate-flavored caramel)	204	49.5	1.1	1.4	6	0
Chocolate-coated peanuts	318	22.2	9.3	23.4	66	1
(chocolate-coated fudge with nuts)	256	38.2	2.8	11.8	41	1
Chocolate-coated raisins	241	40.0	3.1	9.7	36	6
(raisins)	170	44.8	1.8	0.3	2	0
Chocolate-coated vanilla cream	247	39.9	2.2	9.7	35	1
(candy, chocolate-flavored caramel)	204	49.5	1.1	1.4	6	0
Chocolate malt cake	196	37.8	1.9	4.9	23	31
(angel food cake)	153	34.1	4.0	0.1	1	0
Chocolate meringue pie	143	19.0	2.7	6.8	43	35
(low-cal chocolate flavor mousse)	40	5.6	1.4	1.4	31	0
Chocolate syrup, fudge type	196	33.4	2.5	7.6	32	7
(chocolate syrup, thin type)	139	35.6	1.3	1.1	7	0

( ) indicates possible substitute foods that are lower in calories and/or fat.

Serving size--2 ounces:	Calories kcal	Carbo grams	Prot grams	Fat grams	Fat % of kcal	Chol mg
Chocolate syrup, thin type	139	35.6	1.3	1.1	7	0
(low-calorie syrup)	44	11.9	0	0	0	0
Chocolate truffles	276	25.5	3.2	19.4	60	29
(candy, chocolate-flavored caramel)	204	49.5	1.1	1.4	6	0
Coconut custard pie	133	14.1	3.4	7.1	48	58
(low-calorie pudding, prepared)	32	5.6	1.9	0	0	0
Coffee cake	180	29.9	3.1	5.4	27	28
(angel food cake)	153	34.1	4.0	0.1	1	0
Cookies, chocolate	252	40.5	4.0	8.9	32	22
(cookies, fig bars)	197	40.2	2.1	4.1	18	0
Cookies, chocolate chip	273	37.8	3.1	12.8	41	0
(cookies, fig bars)	197	40.2	2.1	4.1	18	0
Cookies, coconut bars	280	36.2	3.5	13.9	45	62
(cookies, fig bars)	197	40.2	2.1	4.1	18	0
Cookies, fig bars	197	40.2	2.1	4.1	18	0
(figs, fresh)	42	10.9	0.5	0.2	4	0
Cookies, gingersnaps	236	43.6	3.2	5.6	21	0
(cookies, fig bars)	197	40.2	2.1	4.1	18	0
Cookies, ladyfingers	207	33.8	6.0	5.2	23	207
(angel food cake)	153	34.1	4.0	0.1	1	0
Cookies, macaroons	229	40.9	2.0	7.2	27	0
(cookies, fig bars)	197	40.2	2.1	4.1	18	0
Cookies, marshmallow	239	38.4	2.3	9.6	35	0
(cookies, fig bars)	197	40.2	2.1	4.1	18	0
Cookies, molasses	244	41.8	3.2	7.3	27	0
(cookies, fig bars)	197	40.2	2.1	4.1	18	0
Cookies, oatmeal with raisins	256	41.7	3.5	8.7	31	22
(cookies, fig bars)	197	40.2	2.1	4.1	18	0
Cookies, peanut butter	269	33.4	5.1	13.5	44	18
(cookies, fig bars)	197	40.2	2.1	4.1	18	0
Cookies, raisin	227	38.5	2.3	7.7	30	1
(raisins)	170	44.8	1.8	0.3	2	0
Cookies, sandwich type	281	39.3	2.7	12.8	41	22
(cookies, fig bars)	197	40.2	2.1	4.1	18	0

( ) indicates possible substitute foods that are lower in calories and/or fat.

Bread

Serving size--2 ounces:	Calories kcal	Carbo grams	Prot grams	Fat grams	Fat % of kcal	Chol mg
Cookies, shortbread	284	36.9	3.5	13.7	44	11
(cookies, fig bars)	197	40.2	2.1	4.1	18	0
Cookies, sugar	271	38.5	2.9	12.0	39	29
(cookies, fig bars)	197	40.2	2.1	4.1	18	0
Cookies, sugar wafers	290	39.7	2.3	13.8	43	0
(cookies, fig bars)	197	40.2	2.1	4.1	18	0
Cookies, thin butter	265	39.0	3.5	9.6	36	49
(cookies, fig bars)	197	40.2	2.1	4.1	18	0
Cookies, vanilla wafers	250	41.7	2.8	8.6	30	33
(cookies, fig bars)	197	40.2	2.1	4.1	18	0
Corn flour	205	43.5	3.9	2.2	9	0
(rye flour, medium)	201	43.9	5.3	1.0	4	0
Corn fritters	214	22.5	4.4	12.2	51	50
(cornmeal, cooked)	28	6.1	0.6	0.1	3	0
Corn muffins	178	27.3	4.0	5.7	29	33
(english muffin, plain)	133	26.1	4.4	1.0	7	0
Corn pone	116	20.5	2.6	3.0	23	2
(cornmeal, cooked)	28	6.1	0.6	0.1	3	0
Corn syrup, light and dark	160	43.4	0	0	0	0
(maple syrup)	148	38.1	0	0.1	1	0
Cornbread	117	16.5	4.2	4.1	32	46
(cornmeal, cooked)	28	6.1	0.6	0.1	3	0
Cornmeal, cooked	28	6.1	0.6	0.1	3	0
(farina, cooked)	14	3.0	0.4	0	0	0
Cornstarch	205	49.7	0.2	0	0	0
(no alternate identified)						
Cracked wheat bread	147	28.0	4.9	2.2	13	0
(low-calorie wheat bread)	100	15.0	5.0	2.1	19	0
Cream puffs	146	13.0	3.8	8.8	54	76
(low-calorie pudding, prepared)	32	5.6	1.9	0	0	0
Croissants	230	25.9	4.6	11.9	47	42
(english muffin, plain)	133	26.1	4.4	1.0	7	0
Cupcake	203	35.6	1.9	6.2	27	41
(plain muffins)	168	23.5	3.9	6.5	35	22

( ) indicates possible substitute foods that are lower in calories and/or fat.

Serving size--2 ounces:	Calories kcal	Carbo grams	Prot grams	Fat grams	Fat % of kcal	Chol mg
Custard, baked	65	6.3	3.1	3.1	43	60
(low-calorie pudding, prepared)	32	5.6	1.9	0	0	0
Custard pie	119	11.8	3.1	6.6	50	19
(low-calorie pudding, prepared)	32	5.6	1.9	0	0	0
Danish, cheese	212	21.1	4.5	12.4	52	25
(angel food cake)	153	34.1	4.0	0.1	1	0
Danish, cinnamon	228	25.3	4	12.7	49	17
(angel food cake)	153	34.1	4.0	0.1	1	0
Danish, fruit	210	27.1	3.1	10.5	44	12
(angel food cake)	153	34.1	4.0	0.1	1	0
Danish pastry	244	25.9	4.2	14.3	52	26
(plain muffins)	168	23.5	3.9	6.5	35	22
Dessert topping, ready to eat	107	9.4	2.0	7.0	59	6
(low-calorie dessert topping)	32	0	0	3.6	100	0
Devil's food cake	210	24.8	2.0	12.4	53	29
(angel food cake)	153	34.1	4.0	0.1	1	0
Doughnuts (donuts), cake type	222	29.1	2.6	10.5	43	34
(bagel, raisin & honey w/cinnamon)	160	32.0	6.4	0.8	4	0
Doughnuts (donuts), glazed	241	28.8	2.9	13.0	48	18
(bagel, raisin & honey w/cinnamon)	160	32.0	6.4	0.8	4	0
Doughnuts (donuts), plain	235	21.4	3.6	15.1	58	14
(bagel, plain)	156	30.3	5.9	0.9	5	0
Doughnuts, cake type	222	29.1	2.6	10.5	43	34
(plain muffins)	168	23.5	3.9	6.5	35	22
Eclairs	148	13.7	3.6	8.9	54	72
(low-calorie pudding, prepared)	32	5.6	1.9	0	0	0
English muffin, plain	133	26.1	4.4	1.0	7	0
(low-calorie rye bread)	108	24.3	5.4	0.7	6	0
French toast	134	20.2	5.2	3.4	23	125
(english muffin, plain)	133	26.1	4.4	1.0	7	0
Frozen dessert topping	180	13.0	0.7	14.3	71	0
(low-calorie dessert topping)	32	0	0	3.6	100	0
Fruitcake, dark	215	33.8	2.7	8.7	36	26
(angel food cake)	153	34.1	4.0	0.1	1	0

( ) indicates possible substitute foods that are lower in calories and/or fat.

Serving size--2 ounces:	Calories kcal	Carbo grams	Prot grams	Fat grams	Fat % of kcal	Chol mg
Fruitcake, light	214	31.9	3.4	8.9	37	15
(angel food cake)	153	34.1	4.0	0.1	1	0
Gelatin dessert, prepared	33	8.0	0.9	0	0	0
(low-calorie gelatin, prepared)	4	0	0.9	0	0	0
Hard candy	211	55.6	0	0	0	0
(candy, marshmallows)	180	46.1	1.0	0.1	0	0
Hard rolls (kaiser rolls)	166	29.9	5.6	2.4	13	0
(low-calorie white bread)	100	17.5	5.0	2.1	19	0
Honey	172	46.7	0.2	0	0	0
(maple syrup)	148	38.1	0	0.1	1	0
Honey spice cake	200	34.5	2.3	6.1	27	33
(angel food cake)	153	34.1	4.0	0.1	1	0
Hostess lights apple spice cakes	174	38.7	2.7	1.4	7	0
(angel food cake)	153	34.1	4.0	0.1	1	0
Hostess lights chocolate cupcakes	174	34.6	2.7	2.7	14	0
(angel food cake)	153	34.1	4.0	0.1	1	0
Hostess lights van pudng choc cake	174	37.3	2.7	1.4	7	0
(angel food cake)	153	34.1	4.0	0.1	1	0
Hostess regular creme filled cakes	200	33.3	2.2	6.7	30	6
(hostess lights chocolate cupcakes)	174	34.6	2.7	2.7	14	0
Hostess twinkies	213	34.6	1.4	8.0	34	13
(hostess twinkies light)	169	32.3	3.1	3.1	17	0
Hostess twinkies light	169	32.3	3.1	3.1	17	0
(angel food cake)	153	34.1	4.0	0.1	1	0
Ice cream cone (without ice cream)	214	44.2	5.7	1.4	6	0
(frozen yogurt, nonfat)	48	10.5	2.0	0	0	0
Ice cream, french vanilla	124	12.5	2.3	7.4	54	50
(ice milk, hard vanilla)	79	12.5	2.2	2.4	27	8
Ice cream, vanilla, 10% fat	115	13.5	2.0	6.1	48	25
(ice milk, hard vanilla)	79	12.5	2.2	2.4	27	8
Ice cream, vanilla, 16% fat	134	12.2	1.6	9.1	61	34
(ice milk, hard vanilla)	79	12.5	2.2	2.4	27	8
Ice milk, hard vanilla	79	12.5	2.2	2.4	27	8
(frozen yogurt, nonfat)	48	10.5	2.0	0	0	0

( ) indicates possible substitute foods that are lower in calories and/or fat.

Serving size--2 ounces:	Calories kcal	Carbo grams	Prot grams	Fat grams	Fat % of kcal	Chol mg
Ice milk, soft vanilla	71	12.4	2.8	1.5	18	7
(frozen yogurt, nonfat)	48	10.5	2.0	0	0	0
Lemon chiffon pie	177	24.8	4.0	7.1	36	96
(lemon meringue pie)	161	22.2	2.2	7.3	40	30
Lemon meringue pie	161	22.2	2.2	7.3	40	30
(low-calorie pudding, prepared)	32	5.6	1.9	0	0	0
M&m's brand plain chocolate candy	295	40.8	4.5	12.5	38	6
(candy, chocolate-flavored caramel)	204	49.5	1.1	1.4	6	0
Maple syrup	148	38.1	0	0.1	1	0
(low-calorie syrup)	44	11.9	0	0	0	0
Maraschino cherries	66	16.7	0.1	0.1	1	0
(cherries, sweet, canned w/water)	26	6.7	0.5	0.1	3	0
Marble cake	197	26.8	2.4	9.6	43	41
(angel food cake)	153	34.1	4.0	0.1	1	0
Matzoh	224	47.4	5.7	0.8	3	0
(bagel, plain)	156	30.3	5.9	0.9	5	0
Mince pie	164	27.2	1.5	6.1	32	0
(low-calorie pudding, prepared)	32	5.6	1.9	0	0	0
Modified pound cake	216	29.8	3.4	9.5	39	65
(angel food cake)	153	34.1	4.0	0.1	1	0
Molasses, cane, light	143	36.9	0	0	0	0
(molasses, cane, medium)	132	34.0	0	0	0	0
Molasses, cane, medium	132	34.0	0	0	0	0
(low-calorie syrup)	44	11.9	0	0	0	0
Muffins, blueberry	161	23.1	3.7	6.1	34	21
(english muffin, plain)	133	26.1	4.4	1.0	7	0
Muffins, bran	156	26.4	3.7	5.2	28	39
(english muffin, plain)	133	26.1	4.4	1.0	7	0
Oat bran	139	37.5	9.8	4.0	26	0
(no alternate identified)						
Old-fashioned pound cake	246	27.1	3.6	13.9	50	65
(angel food cake)	153	34.1	4.0	0.1	1	0
Pancakes	129	16	3.6	5.5	39	33
(bread, boston brown)	120	25.9	3.1	0.7	5	1

( ) indicates possible substitute foods that are lower in calories and/or fat.

Serving size--2 ounces:	Calories kcal	Carbo grams	Prot grams	Fat grams	Fat % of kcal	Chol mg
Peach pie	126	18.6	1.1	5.7	39	0
(peaches, fresh)	24	6.3	0.4	0.1	4	0
Pecan pie	233	29.6	2.8	12.6	47	49
(low-calorie pudding, prepared)	32	5.6	1.9	0	0	0
Pie crust	259	25.0	2.2	16.5	58	0
(apple pie)	150	21.0	1.4	7.1	42	0
Pineapple chiffon pie	163	22.2	3.7	6.9	38	86
(pineapple custard pie)	125	18.2	2.3	4.9	35	35
Pineapple custard pie	125	18.2	2.3	4.9	35	35
(pineapple, fresh)	28	7.0	0.2	0.2	6	0
Pineapple pie	143	21.6	1.2	6.1	38	6
(pineapple, fresh)	28	7.0	0.2	0.2	6	0
Pita bread	156	31.6	5.2	0.7	4	0
(low-calorie rye bread)	108	24.3	5.4	0.7	6	0
Plain muffins	168	23.5	3.9	6.5	35	22
(english muffin, plain)	133	26.1	4.4	1.0	7	0
Pop tarts brown sugar cinnamon	234	36.7	3.3	8.9	34	0
(muffins, blueberry)	161	23.1	3.7	6.1	34	21
Pop tarts frosted blueberry	222	41.1	2.2	5.6	23	0
(muffins, blueberry)	161	23.1	3.7	6.1	34	21
Pop tarts frosted brown sugar cinn	234	37.8	3.3	7.8	30	0
(muffins, blueberry)	161	23.1	3.7	6.1	34	21
Pop tarts frosted ch vanilla creme	222	41.1	3.3	5.6	23	0
(muffins, blueberry)	161	23.1	3.7	6.1	34	21
Pop tarts frosted cherry	222	41.1	2.2	5.6	23	0
(muffins, blueberry)	161	23.1	3.7	6.1	34	21
Pop tarts frosted chocolate fudge	222	41.1	3.3	5.6	23	0
(muffins, blueberry)	161	23.1	3.7	6.1	34	21
Pop tarts frosted dutch apple	234	41.1	2.2	6.7	26	0
(muffins, blueberry)	161	23.1	3.7	6.1	34	21
Pop tarts frosted raspberry	222	41.1	2.2	5.6	23	0
(muffins, blueberry)	161	23.1	3.7	6.1	34	21
Pop tarts frosted strawberry	222	41.1	2.2	5.6	23	0
(muffins, blueberry)	161	23.1	3.7	6.1	34	21

( ) indicates possible substitute foods that are lower in calories and/or fat.

Serving size--2 ounces:	Calories kcal	Carbo grams	Prot grams	Fat grams	Fat % of kcal	Chol mg
Pop tarts milk chocolate	234	41.1	3.3	6.7	26	0
(muffins, blueberry)	161	23.1	3.7	6.1	34	21
Pop tarts strawberry	234	41.1	2.2	6.7	26	0
(muffins, blueberry)	161	23.1	3.7	6.1	34	21
Popovers, baked	124	15.9	4.9	4.3	32	65
(bread, boston brown)	120	25.9	3.1	0.7	5	1
Pressurized dessert topping	150	9.1	0.6	12.6	76	0
(low-calorie dessert topping)	32	0	0	3.6	100	0
Pretzels	216	44.9	5.2	2.0	8	0
(chestnuts, roasted)	138	30.0	1.8	1.2	8	0
Prune whip	88	20.9	2.5	0.1	1	0
(plums, fresh)	31	7.4	0.5	0.3	9	0
Pudding, chocolate	84	14.6	1.8	2.7	29	6
(low-cal chocolate flavor mousse)	40	5.6	1.4	1.4	31	0
Pudding mix, custard, cooked	74	12.8	1.8	2.0	24	7
(low-calorie pudding, prepared)	32	5.6	1.9	0	0	0
Pudding, vanilla	63	9.0	2.0	2.2	31	8
(low-calorie pudding, prepared)	32	5.6	1.9	0	0	0
Pumpkin pie	116	15.0	2.5	5.3	41	24
(low-calorie pudding, prepared)	32	5.6	1.9	0	0	0
Raisin pie	153	24.4	1.5	6.1	36	6
(low-calorie pudding, prepared)	32	5.6	1.9	0	0	0
Rhubarb pie	143	21.7	1.4	6.1	38	0
(low-calorie pudding, prepared)	32	5.6	1.9	0	0	0
Rice pudding with raisins	83	15.1	2.0	1.8	20	6
(low-calorie pudding, prepared)	32	5.6	1.9	0	0	0
Rolls and buns, plain	169	30.1	4.6	3.2	17	3
(low-calorie white bread)	100	17.5	5.0	2.1	19	0
Rolls and buns, raisin	156	32.0	3.9	1.6	9	2
(bread, boston brown)	120	25.9	3.1	0.7	5	1
Rye flour, medium	198	42.4	6.5	1.0	5	0
(oat bran)	139	37.5	9.8	4.0	26	0
Salt-rising bread	151	29.6	4.5	1.4	8	1
(low-calorie white bread)	100	17.5	5.0	2.1	19	0

( ) indicates possible substitute foods that are lower in calories and/or fat.

Serving size--2 ounces:	Calories kcal	Carbo grams	Prot grams	Fat grams	Fat % of kcal	Chol mg
Salt sticks	218	42.7	6.8	1.6	7	2
(rolls and buns, plain)	169	30.1	4.6	3.2	17	3
Sherbert	79	17.2	0.6	1.1	13	4
(frozen yogurt, nonfat)	48	10.5	2.0	0	0	0
Sorghum syrup	164	42.4	0	0	0	0
(low-calorie syrup)	44	11.9	0	0	0	0
Sponge cake	168	32.7	4.1	2.4	13	96
(angel food cake)	153	34.1	4.0	0.1	1	0
Spoon bread, corn	111	9.6	3.8	6.5	53	73
(cornmeal, cooked)	28	6.1	0.6	0.1	3	0
Strawberry pie	112	17.5	1.1	4.5	36	5
(strawberries, fresh)	17	4.0	0.3	0.2	11	0
Sugar	207	56.4	0	0	0	0
(artificial sweetener)	0	0	0	0	0	0
Sugar-coated almonds	259	39.8	4.4	10.5	36	0
(Sugar-coated popcorn)	217	48.4	3.5	2.0	8	0
Sugar-coated popcorn	217	48.4	3.5	2.0	8	0
(candy, marshmallows)	180	46.1	1.0	0.1	0	0
Sweet potato pie	121	13.4	2.6	6.4	48	31
(low-calorie pudding, prepared)	32	5.6	1.9	0	0	0
Sweet rolls	211	28.8	3.5	9.3	39	37
(english muffin, plain)	133	26.1	4.4	1.0	7	0
Tapioca, apple, dessert	66	16.7	0.1	0.1	1	0
(low-calorie pudding, prepared)	32	5.6	1.9	0	0	0
Tapioca, cream pudding	71	9.6	2.7	2.4	31	46
(tapioca, apple, dessert)	66	16.7	0.1	0.1	1	0
Toast with butter and jelly	197	31.3	4.1	6.1	28	14
(english muffin, plain)	133	26.1	4.4	1.0	7	0
Vinegar	8	3.3	0	0	0	0
(no alternate identified)						
Waffles	165	18.6	4.5	8.0	44	39
(english muffin, plain)	133	26.1	4.4	1.0	7	0
Wheat flour, all-purpose	206	43.1	6.0	0.6	3	0
(whole-grain rye)	189	41.6	6.9	1.0	5	0

( ) indicates possible substitute foods that are lower in calories and/or fat.

Serving size--2 ounces:	Calories kcal	Carbo grams	Prot grams	Fat grams	Fat % of kcal	Chol mg
Wheat flour, self-rising	200	42.1	5.3	0.6	3	0
(whole-grain rye)	189	41.6	6.9	1.0	5	0
Wheat germ, crude	206	26.5	15.1	6.2	27	0
(oat bran)	139	37.5	9.8	4.0	26	0
White cake, no icing	173	31.4	2.3	4.4	23	0
(angel food cake)	153	34.1	4.0	0.1	1	0
White cake with coconut icing	210	34.4	2.1	7.5	32	1
(angel food cake)	153	34.1	4.0	0.1	1	0
White cake with white icing	202	35.3	2.2	6.7	30	19
(angel food cake)	153	34.1	4.0	0.1	1	0
Whole-grain rye	189	41.6	6.9	1.0	5	0
(oat bran)	139	37.5	9.8	4.0	26	0
Whole wheat rolls	151	29.0	4.9	2.7	15	0
(low-calorie wheat bread)	100	15.0	5.0	2.1	19	0
Yellow cake, no icing	181	30.8	2.7	5.3	26	33
(angel food cake)	153	34.1	4.0	0.1	1	0
Yellow cake with caramel icing	197	34.5	2.3	6.1	28	40
(angel food cake)	153	34.1	4.0	0.1	1	0
Yellow cake with chocolate icing	207	34.2	2.4	7.4	32	25
(angel food cake)	153	34.1	4.0	0.1	1	0

( ) indicates possible substitute foods that are lower in calories and/or fat.

BREAKFAST CEREAL

Foods in this category have been assigned a serving size of 1 ounce. A small bowl of cold cereal like corn or bran or wheat flakes, without milk, weighs approximately 1 ounce. Ready-to-eat breakfast cereals with dried fruit weigh significantly more, while puffed cereals (puffed rice, puffed corn) generally weigh less. Keep in mind that the nutritional content of breakfast cereals listed in this category does not include milk. See the Dairy Products and Eggs category for comparisons of skim versus low-fat versus whole milk.

Cereal

Hot cereals (e.g., oatmeal, farina, etc.) weigh significantly more than cold cereals. Therefore, to compare one bowl of hot cereal to one bowl of cold cereal, you must multiply the values of the hot cereal by a factor of approximately eight. Also, when comparing hot versus cold cereal, don't forget to include the calories, carbohydrates, protein, fat and cholesterol for any milk you put on your cold cereal!

Weights and Measures

1. One bowl of corn flakes (1 cup) weighs approximately one ounce.
2. One bowl of raisin bran (1 cup) weighs approximately two ounces.
3. One bowl of cooked oatmeal, grits or farina (1 cup) weighs approximately eight ounces.

Serving size--1 ounce:	Calories kcal	Carbo grams	Prot grams	Fat grams	Fat % of kcal	Chol mg
100% bran cereal	76	20.7	3.5	1.4	17	0
(fiber one cereal)	60	21.0	4.0	1.0	15	0
100% natural cereal, plain	133	17.8	3.3	6.1	41	0
(kellogg's raisin bran cereal)	88	21.4	3.1	0.6	5	0
100% natural w/apple & cinn cereal	130	19.0	2.9	5.3	37	0
(kellogg's raisin bran cereal)	88	21.4	3.1	0.6	5	0
100% natural w/raisin & dates cereal	128	18.7	2.9	5.2	37	0
(kellogg's raisin bran cereal)	88	21.4	3.1	0.6	5	0
All-bran	71	21.1	4.1	0.5	6	0
(fiber one cereal)	60	21.0	4.0	1.0	15	0
Almond delight cereal	110	23.0	2.0	2.0	16	0
(kellogg's raisin bran cereal)	88	21.4	3.1	0.6	5	0

( ) indicates possible substitute foods that are lower in calories and/or fat.

Serving size--1 ounce:	Calories kcal	Carbo grams	Prot grams	Fat grams	Fat % of kcal	Chol mg
Alpha-bits cereal	111	24.6	2.2	0.7	6	0
(kellogg's raisin bran cereal)	88	21.4	3.1	0.6	5	0
Apple cinnamon squares cereal	90	23.0	2.0	0	0	0
(all-bran)	71	21.1	4.1	0.5	6	0
Apple fruit wheats cereal	100	23.0	2.0	0	0	0
(kellogg's raisin bran cereal)	88	21.4	3.1	0.6	5	0
Apple jacks cereal	110	25.7	1.5	0.1	1	0
(apple cinnamon squares cereal)	90	23.0	2.0	0	0	0
Apple raisin crisp cereal	100	24.6	1.5	0	0	0
(apple cinnamon squares cereal)	90	23.0	2.0	0	0	0
Bran buds cereal	73	21.5	3.9	0.7	9	0
(fiber one cereal)	60	21.0	4.0	1.0	15	0
Bran chex cereal	90	22.6	2.9	0.8	8	0
(all-bran)	71	21.1	4.1	0.5	6	0
C.w. post, plain cereal	126	20.3	2.6	4.4	31	0
(fruitful bran cereal)	84	22.3	2.3	0	0	0
C.w. post w/raisins cereal	123	20.4	2.4	4.1	30	0
(fruitful bran cereal)	84	22.3	2.3	0	0	0
Cap'n crunch cereal	119	22.9	1.4	2.6	20	0
(apple jacks cereal)	110	25.7	1.5	0.1	1	0
Cap'n crunch crunchberries cereal	118	23.1	1.5	2.4	18	0
(apple jacks cereal)	110	25.7	1.5	0.1	1	0
Cap'n crunch peanut butter cereal	124	21.5	2.0	3.7	27	0
(apple jacks cereal)	110	25.7	1.5	0.1	1	0
Cheerios cereal	111	19.6	4.3	1.8	15	0
(fiber one cereal)	60	21.0	4.0	1.0	15	0
Chocolate chip cookie crisp cereal	110	25.0	1.0	1.0	8	0
(fruitful bran cereal)	84	22.3	2.3	0	0	0
Clusters cereal	100	19.0	3.0	3.0	27	0
(fruitful bran cereal)	84	22.3	2.3	0	0	0
Cocoa krispies cereal	110	25.2	1.5	0.4	3	0
(fruitful bran cereal)	84	22.3	2.3	0	0	0
Cocoa pebbles cereal	116	24.4	1.3	1.5	12	0
(fruitful bran cereal)	84	22.3	2.3	0	0	0

( ) indicates possible substitute foods that are lower in calories and/or fat.

Serving size--1 ounce:	Calories kcal	Carbo grams	Prot grams	Fat grams	Fat % of kcal	Chol mg
Cookiecrisp cereal	113	24.8	1.4	1.0	8	0
(kellogg's raisin bran cereal)	88	21.4	3.1	0.6	5	0
Corn bran cereal	98	23.9	1.9	1.0	9	0
(kellogg's raisin bran cereal)	88	21.4	3.1	0.6	5	0
Corn chex cereal	111	24.9	2.0	0.1	1	0
(kellogg's raisin bran cereal)	88	21.4	3.1	0.6	5	0
Corn pops cereal	110	26.0	1.0	0	0	0
(kellogg's raisin bran cereal)	88	21.4	3.1	0.6	5	0
Count chocula cereal	110	24.0	2.0	1.0	8	0
(kellogg's raisin bran cereal)	88	21.4	3.1	0.6	5	0
Cracklin' bran cereal	108	19.4	2.6	4.1	34	0
(all-bran)	71	21.1	4.1	0.5	6	0
Cracklin' oat bran cereal	110	20.0	3.0	4.0	33	0
(all-bran)	71	21.1	4.1	0.5	6	0
Cream of rice, cooked	15	3.3	0.3	0	0	0
(farina, cooked)	14	3.0	0.4	0	0	0
Cream of wheat, regular, cooked	15	3.1	0.4	0.1	6	0
(farina, cooked)	14	3.0	0.4	0	0	0
Crispix cereal	110	25.0	2.0	0	0	0
(apple cinnamon squares cereal)	90	23.0	2.0	0	0	0
Crispy critters cereal	110	24.0	2.0	1.0	8	0
(apple cinnamon squares cereal)	90	23.0	2.0	0	0	0
Crispy rice cereal	112	25.1	1.8	0.1	1	0
(apple cinnamon squares cereal)	90	23.0	2.0	0	0	0
Crispy wheats 'n raisins cereal	99	23.1	2.0	0.5	4	0
(kellogg's raisin squares cereal)	90	22.0	2.0	0	0	0
Crunchy nut oh!s cereal	130	20.0	2.0	4.0	28	0
(kellogg's raisin bran cereal)	88	21.4	3.1	0.6	5	0
Farina, cooked	14	3.0	0.4	0	0	0
(no alternate identified)						
Fiber one cereal	60	21.0	4.0	1.0	15	0
(no alternate identified)						
Frosted mini-wheats cereal	102	23.4	2.9	0.3	3	0
(apple cinnamon squares cereal)	90	23.0	2.0	0	0	0

( ) indicates possible substitute foods that are lower in calories and/or fat.

Serving size--1 ounce:	Calories kcal	Carbo grams	Prot grams	Fat grams	Fat % of kcal	Chol mg
Frosted rice krinkles cereal	109	25.8	1.4	0.1	1	0
(apple cinnamon squares cereal)	90	23.0	2.0	0	0	0
Frosted rice krispies cereal	109	25.7	1.4	0.1	1	0
(apple cinnamon squares cereal)	90	23.0	2.0	0	0	0
Fruit islands cereal	110	26.0	1.0	0	0	0
(kellogg's raisin bran cereal)	88	21.4	3.1	0.6	5	0
Fruit loops cereal	111	25.0	1.7	0.5	4	0
(kellogg's raisin bran cereal)	88	21.4	3.1	0.6	5	0
Fruitful bran cereal	88	23.0	2.0	1	10	0
(all-bran)	71	21.1	4.1	0.5	6	0
Fruity marshmallow krispies	108	24.6	1.5	0	0	0
(kellogg's raisin bran cereal)	88	21.4	3.1	0.6	5	0
Fruity pebbles cereal	115	24.4	1.1	1.5	12	0
(kellogg's raisin bran cereal)	88	21.4	3.1	0.6	5	0
Golden grahams cereal	109	24.1	1.6	1.1	9	0
(apple cinnamon squares cereal)	90	23.0	2.0	0	0	0
Graham crackos cereal	102	24.5	2.1	0.2	2	0
(apple cinnamon squares cereal)	90	23.0	2.0	0	0	0
Granola	138	15.6	3.6	7.7	50	0
(apple cinnamon squares cereal)	90	23.0	2.0	0	0	0
Grape-nuts cereal	101	23.2	3.3	0.1	1	0
(fiber one cereal)	60	21.0	4.0	1.0	15	0
Grape-nuts flakes cereal	101	23.2	3.0	0.3	3	0
(fiber one cereal)	60	21.0	4.0	1.0	15	0
Grits, white, cooked	17	3.7	0.4	0.1	5	0
(farina, cooked)	14	3.0	0.4	0	0	0
Heartland natural cereal, plain	123	19.4	2.9	4.4	32	0
(fiber one cereal)	60	21.0	4.0	1.0	15	0
Heartland natural w/coconut cereal	125	19.2	2.9	4.6	33	0
(fiber one cereal)	60	21.0	4.0	1.0	15	0
Heartland natural w/raisin cereal	120	19.6	2.7	4.0	30	0
(fiber one cereal)	60	21.0	4.0	1.0	15	0
Honey and nut corn flakes	113	23.3	1.8	1.6	13	0
(fiber one cereal)	60	21.0	4.0	1.0	15	0

( ) indicates possible substitute foods that are lower in calories and/or fat.

Serving size--1 ounce:	Calories kcal	Carbo grams	Prot grams	Fat grams	Fat % of kcal	Chol mg
Honey bran cereal	97	23.2	2.5	0.6	6	0
(all-bran)	71	21.1	4.1	0.5	6	0
Honey graham chex cereal	110	25.0	1.0	1.0	8	0
(apple cinnamon squares cereal)	90	23.0	2.0	0	0	0
Honey graham oh!s cereal	130	21.0	1.0	4.0	28	0
(apple cinnamon squares cereal)	90	23.0	2.0	0	0	0
Honey nut cheerios cereal	107	22.8	3.1	0.7	6	0
(apple cinnamon squares cereal)	90	23.0	2.0	0	0	0
Honeycomb cereal	111	25.3	1.6	0.5	4	0
(apple cinnamon squares cereal)	90	23.0	2.0	0	0	0
Instant corn grits, plain, cooked	17	3.7	0.4	0	0	0
(farina, cooked)	14	3.0	0.4	0	0	0
Instant cream of wheat, cooked	18	3.7	0.5	0.1	5	0
(farina, cooked)	14	3.0	0.4	0	0	0
Instant oats, plain, cooked	17	2.9	0.7	0.3	16	0
(farina, cooked)	14	3.0	0.4	0	0	0
Just right cereal	100	22.3	2.3	0.8	7	0
(all-bran)	71	21.1	4.1	0.5	6	0
Kellogg's sugar frosted flakes cereal	108	25.7	1.4	0.1	1	0
(all-bran)	71	21.1	4.1	0.5	6	0
Kellogg's 40% bran flakes cereal	92	22.2	3.6	0.5	5	0
(all-bran)	71	21.1	4.1	0.5	6	0
Kellogg's bran flakes cereal	90	23.0	3.0	0	0	0
(all-bran)	71	21.1	4.1	0.5	6	0
Kellogg's corn flakes cereal	110	24.4	2.3	0.1	1	0
(kellogg's raisin bran cereal)	88	21.4	3.1	0.6	5	0
Kellogg's raisin bran cereal	88	21.4	3.1	0.6	5	0
(all-bran)	71	21.1	4.1	0.5	6	0
Kellogg's raisin squares cereal	90	22.0	2.0	0	0	0
(all-bran)	71	21.1	4.1	0.5	6	0
King vitaman cereal	115	24.1	1.5	1.6	13	0
(all-bran)	71	21.1	4.1	0.5	6	0
Kix cereal	110	23.4	2.6	0.7	6	0
(all-bran)	71	21.1	4.1	0.5	6	0

( ) indicates possible substitute foods that are lower in calories and/or fat.

Serving size--1 ounce:	Calories kcal	Carbo grams	Prot grams	Fat grams	Fat % of kcal	Chol mg
Life, plain/cinnamon cereal	105	20.3	5.2	0.5	4	0
(apple cinnamon squares cereal)	90	23.0	2.0	0	0	0
Lucky charms cereal	111	23.2	2.6	1.1	9	0
(kellogg's raisin bran cereal)	88	21.4	3.1	0.6	5	0
Malt-o-meal, cooked	14	3.1	0.4	0	0	0
(no alternate identified)						
Maltex, cooked	20	4.5	0.7	0.1	4	0
(malt-o-meal, cooked)	14	3.1	0.4	0	0	0
Maypo, cooked	20	3.8	0.7	0.3	13	0
(malt-o-meal, cooked)	14	3.1	0.4	0	0	0
Most cereal	96	21.6	4.0	0.3	3	0
(all-bran)	71	21.1	4.1	0.5	6	0
Natural valley granola cereal	126	18.9	2.9	4.9	35	0
(apple cinnamon squares cereal)	90	23.0	2.0	0	0	0
Nut & honey crunch cereal	110	24.0	2.0	1.0	8	0
(apple cinnamon squares cereal)	90	23.0	2.0	0	0	0
Nutri-grain cereal, barley	105	23.5	3.1	0.2	2	0
(kellogg's raisin bran cereal)	88	21.4	3.1	0.6	5	0
Nutri-grain cereal, corn	108	23.9	2.3	0.7	6	0
(all-bran)	71	21.1	4.1	0.5	6	0
Nutri-grain cereal, rye	102	24.0	2.5	0.2	2	0
(kellogg's raisin bran cereal)	88	21.4	3.1	0.6	5	0
Nutri-grain cereal, wheat	102	24.0	2.5	0.3	3	0
(kellogg's raisin bran cereal)	88	21.4	3.1	0.6	5	0
Nutri-grain nuggets cereal	100	23.0	3.0	1.0	9	0
(all-bran)	71	21.1	4.1	0.5	6	0
Nutrific cereal	93	22.1	2.2	0.7	7	0
(kellogg's raisin bran cereal)	88	21.4	3.1	0.6	5	0
Oatmeal, cooked	18	3.1	0.7	0.3	15	0
(farina, cooked)	14	3.0	0.4	0	0	0
Oatmeal raisin crisp cereal	110	21.0	2.0	2.0	16	0
(kellogg's raisin squares cereal)	90	22.0	2.0	0	0	0
Post fruit and fiber cereal	90	22.0	2.0	1.0	10	0
(all-bran)	71	21.1	4.1	0.5	6	0

( ) indicates possible substitute foods that are lower in calories and/or fat.

Serving size--1 ounce:	Calories kcal	Carbo grams	Prot grams	Fat grams	Fat % of kcal	Chol mg
Pro grain cereal	100	24.0	3.0	0	0	0
(kellogg's raisin bran cereal)	88	21.4	3.1	0.6	5	0
Product 19 cereal	108	23.5	2.8	0.2	2	0
(all-bran)	71	21.1	4.1	0.5	6	0
Puffed rice cereal	114	25.5	1.8	0.1	1	0
(apple cinnamon squares cereal)	90	23.0	2.0	0	0	0
Puffed wheat cereal	103	22.6	4.2	0.3	3	0
(apple cinnamon squares cereal)	90	23.0	2.0	0	0	0
Quaker oats apple/cinnamon cooked	26	5.0	0.7	0.3	10	0
(quaker oats, brn sugar/raisn, cooked)	23	4.4	0.7	0.3	12	0
Quaker oats, brn sugar/raisn, cooked	23	4.4	0.7	0.3	12	0
(instant oats, plain, cooked)	17	2.9	0.7	0.3	16	0
Quaker oats, cinn/spice, cooked	31	6.2	0.9	0.3	9	0
(quaker oats, brn sugar/raisn, cooked)	23	4.4	0.7	0.3	12	0
Quaker oats, maple/sugar, cooked	30	5.8	0.9	0.3	9	0
(quaker oats, brn sugar/raisn, cooked)	23	4.4	0.7	0.3	12	0
Quaker oats, rais/spice, cooked	29	5.7	0.8	0.3	9	0
(quaker oats, brn sugar/raisn, cooked)	23	4.4	0.7	0.3	12	0
Quisp cereal	117	23.6	1.4	2.0	15	0
(apple cinnamon squares cereal)	90	23.0	2.0	0	0	0
Raisin fruit wheats cereal	100	23.0	2.0	0	0	0
(kellogg's raisin squares cereal)	90	22.0	2.0	0	0	0
Raisin nut bran cereal	110	21.0	2.0	3.0	25	0
(all-bran)	71	21.1	4.1	0.5	6	0
Raisins, rice and rye cereal	95	24.2	1.6	0.1	1	0
(kellogg's raisin bran cereal)	88	21.4	3.1	0.6	5	0
Rice chex cereal	112	25.3	1.5	0.1	1	0
(apple cinnamon squares cereal)	90	23.0	2.0	0	0	0
Rice krispies cereal	112	24.8	1.9	0.2	2	0
(apple cinnamon squares cereal)	90	23.0	2.0	0	0	0
Shreaded wheat cereal, large biscuit	100	22.6	3.1	0.4	4	0
(all-bran)	71	21.1	4.1	0.5	6	0
Shreaded wheat cereal, small biscuit	102	22.6	3.1	0.6	5	0
(apple cinnamon squares cereal)	90	23.0	2.0	0	0	0

( ) indicates possible substitute foods that are lower in calories and/or fat.

Serving size--1 ounce:	Calories kcal	Carbo grams	Prot grams	Fat grams	Fat % of kcal	Chol mg
Special k cereal	111	21.3	5.6	0.1	1	0
(kellogg's raisin bran cereal)	88	21.4	3.1	0.6	5	0
Strawberry fruit wheats cereal	100	23.0	2.0	0	0	0
(kellogg's raisin bran cereal)	88	21.4	3.1	0.6	5	0
Sugar corn pops cereal	108	25.7	1.4	0.1	1	0
(apple cinnamon squares cereal)	90	23.0	2.0	0	0	0
Sugar smacks cereal	106	24.7	2.0	0.5	4	0
(apple cinnamon squares cereal)	90	23.0	2.0	0	0	0
Sun flakes cereal	110	24.0	2.0	1.0	8	0
(all-bran)	71	21.1	4.1	0.5	6	0
Super golden crisp cereal	110	26.0	2.0	0	0	0
(apple cinnamon squares cereal)	90	23.0	2.0	0	0	0
Super sugar crisp cereal	106	25.6	1.8	0.3	3	0
(apple cinnamon squares cereal)	90	23.0	2.0	0	0	0
Tasteeos cereal	111	22.4	3.6	0.8	6	0
(all-bran)	71	21.1	4.1	0.5	6	0
Team cereal	111	24.3	1.8	0.5	4	0
(all-bran)	71	21.1	4.1	0.5	6	0
Toasted oats cereal	110	20.0	4.0	2.0	16	0
(all-bran)	71	21.1	4.1	0.5	6	0
Toasties cereal	110	24.3	2.3	0.1	1	0
(apple cinnamon squares cereal)	90	23.0	2.0	0	0	0
Total cereal	100	22.3	2.8	0.6	5	0
(all-bran)	71	21.1	4.1	0.5	6	0
Trix cereal	109	25.2	1.5	0.4	3	0
(apple cinnamon squares cereal)	90	23.0	2.0	0	0	0
Uncle sam cereal	110	19.0	4.0	2.0	16	0
(all-bran)	71	21.1	4.1	0.5	6	0
Waffelos cereal	115	24.5	1.6	1.2	9	0
(all-bran)	71	21.1	4.1	0.5	6	0
Wheat 'n raisin chex cereal	97	22.6	2.7	0.2	2	0
(kellogg's raisin bran cereal)	88	21.4	3.1	0.6	5	0
Wheat chex cereal	104	23.3	2.8	0.7	6	0
(apple cinnamon squares cereal)	90	23.0	2.0	0	0	0

( ) indicates possible substitute foods that are lower in calories and/or fat.

Serving size--1 ounce:	Calories kcal	Carbo grams	Prot grams	Fat grams	Fat % of kcal	Chol mg
Wheat germ, toasted, plain cereal	108	14.1	8.2	3.0	25	0
(fiber one cereal)	60	21.0	4.0	1.0	15	0
Wheat germ, toasted w/sugar, cereal	107	17.2	6.2	2.3	19	0
(fiber one cereal)	60	21.0	4.0	1.0	15	0
Wheatena, cooked	16	3.3	0.6	0.1	6	0
(farina, cooked)	14	3.0	0.4	0	0	0
Wheaties cereal	99	22.5	2.7	0.5	5	0
(all-bran)	71	21.1	4.1	0.5	6	0
Whole wheat natural cereal, cooked	18	3.9	0.6	0.1	5	0
(cream of wheat, regular, cooked)	15	3.1	0.4	0.1	6	0

( ) indicates possible substitute foods that are lower in calories and/or fat.

CHIPS, CRACKERS, NUTS & SEEDS

The serving size for this category is 1 ounce. In addition to the fact that 1 ounce is an appropriate serving size for most of the items in this category, it is an exceptionally easy figure to convert to other serving sizes for comparisons with foods in other categories.

Weights and Measures

1. Fourteen potato chips (2/32" to 3/32" thick, 1.75" x 2.5") weigh approximately one ounce.
2. Thirty Virginia type peanuts, without shells, weigh approximately one ounce.
3. Eighteen medium-size cashews weigh approximately one ounce.
4. Ten saltine crackers (1 7/8" square, 1/8" thick) weigh approximately one ounce.
5. One graham cracker (5" x 2.5" x 3/16") weighs approximately one-half ounce.

Serving size--1 ounce:	Calories kcal	Carbo grams	Prot grams	Fat grams	Fat % of kcal	Chol mg
Almond butter	179	6.0	4.3	16.8	84	0
(cashew butter)	166	7.8	5.0	14.0	76	0
Almond paste	126	12.3	3.3	7.7	55	0
(no alternate identified)						
Almonds, dried, blanched	166	5.2	5.8	14.9	81	0
(chestnuts, roasted)	69	15.0	0.9	0.6	8	0
Almonds, dry roasted	166	6.9	4.6	14.6	79	0
(chestnuts, roasted)	69	15.0	0.9	0.6	8	0
Almonds, oil roasted	175	4.5	5.8	16.4	84	0
(chestnuts, roasted)	69	15.0	0.9	0.6	8	0
Animal crackers	126	21.0	2.0	3.9	28	0
(pretzels)	108	22.4	2.6	1.0	8	0
Beechnuts, dried	163	9.5	1.8	14.2	78	0
(chestnuts, roasted)	69	15.0	0.9	0.6	8	0
Black walnuts, dried	172	3.4	6.9	16.0	84	0
(chestnuts, roasted)	69	15.0	0.9	0.6	8	0

( ) indicates possible substitute foods that are lower in calories and/or fat.

Chips

Serving size--1 ounce:	Calories kcal	Carbo grams	Prot grams	Fat grams	Fat % of kcal	Chol mg
Brazil nuts, dried	186	3.6	4.1	18.8	91	0
(chestnuts, roasted)	69	15.0	0.9	0.6	8	0
Breadfruit seeds, raw	54	8.3	2.1	1.6	27	0
(lotus seeds, raw)	25	4.9	1.2	0.1	4	0
Breadfruit seeds, roasted	59	11.4	1.8	0.8	12	0
(lotus seeds, raw)	25	4.9	1.2	0.1	4	0
Butter crackers	130	19.1	2.0	5.0	35	0
(pretzels)	108	22.4	2.6	1.0	8	0
Butternuts, dried	174	3.4	7.1	16.2	84	0
(chestnuts, roasted)	69	15.0	0.9	0.6	8	0
Cashew butter	166	7.8	5.0	14.0	76	0
(grape jelly)	77	20.0	0	0	0	0
Cashews, dry roasted	163	9.3	4.3	13.1	72	0
(chestnuts, roasted)	69	15.0	0.9	0.6	8	0
Cashews, oil roasted	163	8.1	4.6	13.7	76	0
(chestnuts, roasted)	69	15.0	0.9	0.6	8	0
Cheese crackers	142	16.5	2.9	7.2	46	9
(pretzels)	108	22.4	2.6	1.0	8	0
Cheese puffs/cheese curls	162	15.2	2.0	10.1	56	1
(pretzels)	108	22.4	2.6	1.0	8	0
Cheetos cheese flavored snack	160	15.0	2.0	10.0	56	0
(cheetos light)	140	19.0	2.0	6.0	39	0
Cheetos light	140	19.0	2.0	6.0	39	0
(pretzels)	108	22.4	2.6	1.0	8	0
Cheez-it snack crackers	140	14.0	2.0	8.0	51	0
(pretzels)	108	22.4	2.6	1.0	8	0
Chestnuts, roasted	69	15.0	0.9	0.6	8	0
(lotus seeds, raw)	25	4.9	1.2	0.1	4	0
Chia seeds, dried	134	13.6	4.7	7.5	50	0
(chestnuts, roasted)	69	15.0	0.9	0.6	8	0
Coconut meat, raw	100	4.3	0.9	9.5	85	0
(pineapple, fresh)	14	3.5	0.1	0.1	6	0
Corn chips	152	16.2	2.0	9.1	54	0
(pretzels)	108	22.4	2.6	1.0	8	0

( ) indicates possible substitute foods that are lower in calories and/or fat.

Serving size--1 ounce:	Calories kcal	Carbo grams	Prot grams	Fat grams	Fat % of kcal	Chol mg
Crackers, saltines	123	20.3	2.6	3.4	25	0
(pretzels)	108	22.4	2.6	1.0	8	0
Crackers, sandwich type	139	15.9	4.3	6.8	44	5
(pretzels)	108	22.4	2.6	1.0	8	0
Doritos brand tortilla chips	140	19.0	2.0	7.0	45	0
(nacho cheese doritos light)	122	20.0	2.2	4.5	33	0
English walnuts, dried	182	5.2	4.1	17.5	87	0
(chestnuts, roasted)	69	15.0	0.9	0.6	8	0
Filberts, dried	179	4.3	3.7	17.7	89	0
(chestnuts, roasted)	69	15.0	0.9	0.6	8	0
Filberts, dried, blanched	191	4.5	3.6	19.1	90	0
(chestnuts, roasted)	69	15.0	0.9	0.6	8	0
Filberts, dry roasted	188	5.1	2.8	18.8	90	0
(chestnuts, roasted)	69	15.0	0.9	0.6	8	0
Filberts, oil roasted	187	5.4	4.1	18.0	87	0
(chestnuts, roasted)	69	15.0	0.9	0.6	8	0
Fritos brand corn chips	150	16.0	2.0	10.0	60	0
(pretzels)	108	22.4	2.6	1.0	8	0
Ginkgo nuts, dried	99	20.5	2.9	0.6	5	0
(chestnuts, roasted)	69	15.0	0.9	0.6	8	0
Ginkgo nuts, raw	52	10.7	1.2	0.5	9	0
(lotus seeds, raw)	25	4.9	1.2	0.1	4	0
Graham crackers, chocolate-coated	135	19.2	1.4	6.7	45	0
(graham crackers, plain)	109	20.8	2.3	2.7	22	0
Graham crackers, honey-coated	117	21.7	1.9	3.2	25	0
(graham crackers, plain)	109	20.8	2.3	2.7	22	0
Graham crackers, plain	109	20.8	2.3	2.7	22	0
(cookies, fig bars)	99	20.1	1.0	2.1	18	0
Hi ho crackers	160	16.0	2.0	10.0	56	1
(pretzels)	108	22.4	2.6	1.0	8	0
Hickory nuts	186	5.2	3.6	18.3	89	0
(chestnuts, roasted)	69	15.0	0.9	0.6	8	0
Lay's brand potato chips	150	14.0	2.0	10.0	60	0
(pretzels)	108	22.4	2.6	1.0	8	0

( ) indicates possible substitute foods that are lower in calories and/or fat.

Serving size--1 ounce:	Calories kcal	Carbo grams	Prot grams	Fat grams	Fat % of kcal	Chol mg
Lotus seeds, dried	94	18.3	4.4	0.6	6	0
(lotus seeds, raw)	25	4.9	1.2	0.1	4	0
Lotus seeds, raw	25	4.9	1.2	0.1	4	0
(no alternate identified)						
Macadamia nuts, dried	199	3.9	2.4	20.9	95	0
(chestnuts, roasted)	69	15.0	0.9	0.6	8	0
Macadamia nuts, oil roasted	204	3.7	2.1	21.7	96	0
(chestnuts, roasted)	69	15.0	0.9	0.6	8	0
Matzoh	112	23.7	2.8	0.4	3	0
(bagel, plain)	76	15.2	3.0	0.5	6	0
Mixed nuts, dry roasted	168	7.2	4.9	14.6	78	0
(chestnuts, roasted)	69	15.0	0.9	0.6	8	0
Mixed nuts, oil roasted	174	6.3	4.4	15.9	82	0
(chestnuts, roasted)	69	15.0	0.9	0.6	8	0
Nabisco bacon flavored thins	140	18.0	2.0	8.0	51	3
(pretzels)	108	22.4	2.6	1.0	8	0
Nabisco better cheddar crackers	140	16.0	4.0	8.0	51	3
(pretzels)	108	22.4	2.6	1.0	8	0
Nabisco cheese ritz bits crackers	140	18.0	2.0	8.0	51	3
(pretzels)	108	22.4	2.6	1.0	8	0
Nabisco cheese tid bits crackers	140	16.0	2.0	8.0	51	3
(pretzels)	108	22.4	2.6	1.0	8	0
Nabisco chicken in biskit crackers	160	16.0	2.0	10.0	56	3
(pretzels)	108	22.4	2.6	1.0	8	0
Nabisco escort crackers	140	18.0	2.0	8.0	51	0
(pretzels)	108	22.4	2.6	1.0	8	0
Nabisco harvest crisp crackers	120	20.0	2.0	4.0	30	0
(pretzels)	108	22.4	2.6	1.0	8	0
Nabisco meal mates sesame crackers	140	18.0	2.0	6.0	39	0
(pretzels)	108	22.4	2.6	1.0	8	0
Nabisco nips cheese crackers	140	18.0	2.0	6.0	39	3
(pretzels)	108	22.4	2.6	1.0	8	0
Nabisco oat thins crackers	140	20.0	2.0	6.0	39	0
(pretzels)	108	22.4	2.6	1.0	8	0

( ) indicates possible substitute foods that are lower in calories and/or fat.

Serving size--1 ounce:	Calories kcal	Carbo grams	Prot grams	Fat grams	Fat % of kcal	Chol mg
Nabisco premium saltine crackers	120	20.0	2.0	4.0	30	3
(pretzels)	108	22.4	2.6	1.0	8	0
Nabisco ritz bits crackers	140	18.0	2.0	8.0	51	0
(nabisco premium saltine crackers)	120	20.0	2.0	4.0	30	3
Nabisco ritz crackers	140	18.0	2.0	8.0	51	3
(pretzels)	108	22.4	2.6	1.0	8	0
Nabisco royal lunch crackers	120	20.0	2.0	4.0	30	9
(pretzels)	108	22.4	2.6	1.0	8	0
Nabisco soup & oyster crackers	120	20.0	2.0	4.0	30	3
(pretzels)	108	22.4	2.6	1.0	8	0
Nabisco swiss cheese crackers	140	22.0	2.0	6.0	39	3
(pretzels)	108	22.4	2.6	1.0	8	0
Nabisco triscuit wafers	120	20.0	2.0	4.0	30	0
(pretzels)	108	22.4	2.6	1.0	8	0
Nabisco vegetable thins crackers	140	16.0	2.0	8.0	51	3
(pretzels)	108	22.4	2.6	1.0	8	0
Nabisco waverly crackers	140	20.0	2.0	6.0	39	0
(pretzels)	108	22.4	2.6	1.0	8	0
Nabisco wheat premium plus cracker	120	20.0	2.0	4.0	30	0
(pretzels)	108	22.4	2.6	1.0	8	0
Nabisco wheat thins crackers	140	18.0	2.0	6.0	39	0
(pretzels)	108	22.4	2.6	1.0	8	0
Nacho cheese doritos light	122	20.0	2.2	4.5	33	0
(pretzels)	108	22.4	2.6	1.0	8	0
Peanut butter	168	4.5	8.1	14.5	78	0
(grape jelly)	77	20.0	0	0	0	0
Peanuts, boiled	107	4.1	4.4	8.9	75	0
(chestnuts, roasted)	69	15.0	0.9	0.6	8	0
Peanuts, dried	161	4.6	7.3	13.9	78	0
(peanuts, boiled)	107	4.1	4.4	8.9	75	0
Peanuts, oil roasted	164	5.2	7.6	13.9	76	0
(peanuts, boiled)	107	4.1	4.4	8.9	75	0
Pecans, dried	189	5.2	2.2	19.2	91	0
(chestnuts, roasted)	69	15.0	0.9	0.6	8	0

( ) indicates possible substitute foods that are lower in calories and/or fat.

Serving size--1 ounce:	Calories kcal	Carbo grams	Prot grams	Fat grams	Fat % of kcal	Chol mg
Pecans, dry roasted	187	6.3	2.3	18.3	88	0
(chestnuts, roasted)	69	15.0	0.9	0.6	8	0
Pecans, oil roasted	194	4.5	2.0	20.2	94	0
(chestnuts, roasted)	69	15.0	0.9	0.6	8	0
Pili nuts, dried	204	1.1	3.1	22.5	96	0
(chestnuts, roasted)	69	15.0	0.9	0.6	8	0
Pistachio nuts, dried	164	7.0	5.8	13.7	75	0
(chestnuts, roasted)	69	15.0	0.9	0.6	8	0
Pistachio nuts, dry roasted	172	7.8	4.2	15.0	78	0
(chestnuts, roasted)	69	15.0	0.9	0.6	8	0
Popcorn, air-popped, plain	109	21.7	3.6	1.4	12	0
(chestnuts, roasted)	69	15.0	0.9	0.6	8	0
Popcorn, air-popped, with butter	129	16.8	2.8	6.2	43	13
(popcorn, air-popped, plain)	109	21.7	3.6	1.4	12	0
Popcorn, oil-popped, plain	142	16.2	2.5	8	49	0
(popcorn, air-popped, plain)	109	21.7	3.6	1.4	12	0
Potato chips	148	14.7	1.8	10.0	61	0
(pretzels)	108	22.4	2.6	1.0	8	0
Potato sticks	148	15.1	1.9	9.8	60	0
(pretzels)	108	22.4	2.6	1.0	8	0
Pretzels	108	22.4	2.6	1.0	8	0
(chestnuts, roasted)	69	15.0	0.9	0.6	8	0
Pumpkin seeds, dried	153	5.0	6.9	13.0	76	0
(pretzels)	108	22.4	2.6	1.0	8	0
Pumpkin seeds, roasted	148	3.8	9.4	11.9	72	0
(pretzels)	108	22.4	2.6	1.0	8	0
Soda crackers	124	20.0	2.6	3.7	27	0
(pretzels)	108	22.4	2.6	1.0	8	0
Soybean kernel, roasted	128	8.7	10.5	6.8	48	0
(chestnuts, roasted)	69	15.0	0.9	0.6	8	0
Sugar-coated popcorn	109	24.2	1.7	1.0	8	0
(candy, marshmallows)	90	22.8	0.6	0	0	0
Sunflower seed butter	164	7.8	5.6	13.5	74	0
(grape jelly)	77	20.0	0	0	0	0

( ) indicates possible substitute foods that are lower in calories and/or fat.

Serving size--1 ounce:	Calories kcal	Carbo grams	Prot grams	Fat grams	Fat % of kcal	Chol mg
Sunflower seeds, dried	162	5.3	6.5	14.1	78	0
(soybean kernel, roasted)	128	8.7	10.5	6.8	48	0
Sunflower seeds, dry roasted	165	6.8	5.5	14.1	77	0
(soybean kernel, roasted)	128	8.7	10.5	6.8	48	0
Sunflower seeds, oil roasted	174	4.2	6.1	16.3	84	0
(soybean kernel, roasted)	128	8.7	10.5	6.8	48	0
Sunshine animal crackers	120	22.0	2.0	3.0	23	0
(graham crackers, plain)	109	20.8	2.3	2.7	22	0
Sunshine cheddar snack crackers	160	16.0	4.0	8.0	45	6
(pretzels)	108	22.4	2.6	1.0	8	0
Sunshine cinnamon graham crackers	127	19.9	1.8	5.4	38	0
(graham crackers, plain)	109	20.8	2.3	2.7	22	0
Sunshine honey graham crackers	120	20.0	2.0	4.0	30	0
(graham crackers, plain)	109	20.8	2.3	2.7	22	0
Sunshine krispy saltine crackers	120	22.0	2.0	2.0	15	0
(pretzels)	108	22.4	2.6	1.0	8	0
Sunshine oyster & soup crackers	115	19.1	1.9	3.8	30	0
(pretzels)	108	22.4	2.6	1.0	8	0
Sunshine parmesan snack crackers	140	14.0	4.0	8.0	51	3
(pretzels)	108	22.4	2.6	1.0	8	0
Sunshine sesame snack crackers	140	16.0	2.0	8.0	51	0
(pretzels)	108	22.4	2.6	1.0	8	0
Sunshine wheat snack crackers	120	16.0	2.0	6.0	45	0
(pretzels)	108	22.4	2.6	1.0	8	0
Tahini kernels	172	5.1	5.1	16.0	84	0
(soybean kernel, roasted)	128	8.7	10.5	6.8	48	0
Tortilla chips	142	18.2	2.0	8.1	51	0
(pretzels)	108	22.4	2.6	1.0	8	0
Tostitos brand tortilla chips	130	19.0	2.0	6.0	39	0
(pretzels)	108	22.4	2.6	1.0	8	0
Wheat wafers	160	20.0	2.0	8.0	45	0
(pretzels)	108	22.4	2.6	1.0	8	0
Whole wheat crackers	114	19.3	2.4	3.9	31	0
(pretzels)	108	22.4	2.6	1.0	8	0

( ) indicates possible substitute foods that are lower in calories and/or fat.

DAIRY PRODUCTS AND EGGS

The serving size used in this category, Dairy Products and Eggs, is 4 ounces. While some items in this category are typically consumed in smaller quantities (e.g., butter and cheese), all dairy beverages, yogurt, ice cream and many other dairy products are usually consumed in quantities of 4 ounces or more.

Weights and Measures

1. One slice of cheese (3 1/2" x 3 3/8" x 1/8") weighs approximately one ounce.
2. One stick of butter (4 sticks per pound) weighs four ounces.
3. A half cup of milk weighs approximately four ounces.
4. One cup of ice cream weighs approximately five ounces.
5. One large to extra-large egg weighs approximately two ounces.
6. A half cup yogurt weighs approximately four ounces.

Dairy

Serving size--4 ounces:	Calories kcal	Carbo grams	Prot grams	Fat grams	Fat % of kcal	Chol mg
American cheese	425	1.8	25.1	35.5	75	107
(mozzarella cheese, skim)	288	3.2	27.6	18.0	56	66
American cheese food	372	8.3	22.2	27.9	68	72
(mozzarella cheese, skim)	288	3.2	27.6	18.0	56	66
American cheese spread	329	9.9	18.6	24.0	66	63
(mozzarella cheese, skim)	288	3.2	27.6	18.0	56	66
Blue cheese	400	2.6	24.3	32.5	73	85
(feta cheese)	299	4.6	16.1	24.2	73	101
Brick cheese	421	3.2	26.3	33.7	72	107
(feta cheese)	299	4.6	16.1	24.2	73	101
Brie cheese	379	0.5	23.6	31.4	75	113
(camembert cheese)	340	0.6	22.5	27.6	73	82
Butter regular	813	0.1	0.9	92.0	100	248
(promise ultra fat-free margarine)	37	0	0	0	0	0
Butter whipped	813	0.1	0.9	92.0	100	248
(promise ultra fat-free margarine)	37	0	0	0	0	0
Buttermilk	45	5.4	3.7	1.0	20	4
(milk, skim)	40	5.4	3.9	0.2	4	2

( ) indicates possible substitute foods that are lower in calories and/or fat.

Serving size--4 ounces:	Calories kcal	Carbo grams	Prot grams	Fat grams	Fat % of kcal	Chol mg
Camembert cheese	340	0.6	22.5	27.6	73	82
(mozzarella cheese, skim)	288	3.2	27.6	18.0	56	66
Caraway cheese	426	3.5	28.6	33.1	70	105
(mozzarella cheese, skim)	288	3.2	27.6	18.0	56	66
Cheddar cheese	457	1.5	28.2	37.5	74	119
(feta cheese)	299	4.6	16.1	24.2	73	101
Cheese fondue	301	11.3	16.8	20.8	62	254
(cottage cheese, 1% low fat)	82	3.1	14.1	1.1	12	5
Cheshire cheese	439	5.4	26.5	34.7	71	117
(mozzarella cheese, skim)	288	3.2	27.6	18.0	56	66
Chocolate milk, 1% low fat	71	11.8	3.6	1.1	14	3
(milk, skim)	40	5.4	3.9	0.2	4	2
Chocolate milk, 2% low fat	82	11.8	3.6	2.3	25	8
(chocolate milk, 1% low fat)	71	11.8	3.6	1.1	14	3
Chocolate milk whole	94	11.7	3.6	3.9	37	14
(chocolate milk, 1% low fat)	71	11.8	3.6	1.1	14	3
Colby cheese	447	2.9	27.0	36.4	73	108
(mozzarella cheese, skim)	288	3.2	27.6	18.0	56	66
Cold pack american cheese food	375	9.4	22.3	27.8	67	72
(mozzarella cheese, skim)	288	3.2	27.6	18.0	56	66
Cottage cheese, 1% low fat	82	3.1	14.1	1.1	12	5
(yogurt, plain nonfat)	56	8.1	6.0	0	0	0
Cottage cheese, 2% low fat	102	4.1	15.5	2.2	19	10
(cottage cheese, 1% low fat)	82	3.1	14.1	1.1	12	5
Cottage cheese, creamed	117	3.1	14.2	5.1	39	17
(cottage cheese, 1% low fat)	82	3.1	14.1	1.1	12	5
Cottage cheese, creamed, fruit	141	15.1	11.2	3.9	25	13
(cottage cheese, 1% low fat)	82	3.1	14.1	1.1	12	5
Crab meat quiche	280	9.0	10.2	22.7	73	191
(egg beaters with cheese)	130	3.1	14.1	6.0	42	5
Cream cheese	396	3.1	8.5	39.6	90	124
(feta cheese)	299	4.6	16.1	24.2	73	101
Cream cheese, philly fat free	103	6.8	17.1	0	0	17
(promise ultra fat-free margarine)	37	0	0	0	0	0

( ) indicates possible substitute foods that are lower in calories and/or fat.

Serving size--4 ounces:	Calories kcal	Carbo grams	Prot grams	Fat grams	Fat % of kcal	Chol mg
Cream cheese, philly light soft	240	8.1	12.0	20.0	75	40
(cream cheese, philly fat free)	103	6.8	17.1	0	0	17
Dessert topping, ready to eat	214	18.7	4.1	14.1	59	11
(low-calorie dessert topping)	64	0	0	7.1	100	0
Deviled eggs	286	1.6	11.5	25.6	81	521
(potato salad)	162	12.7	3.1	9.3	52	77
Dry curd cottage cheese	96	2.0	19.6	0.5	5	8
(yogurt, plain nonfat)	56	8.1	6.0	0	0	0
Duck eggs, whole	210	1.6	14.5	15.6	67	1002
(egg beaters)	51	2.0	10.3	0	0	0
Edam cheese	405	1.6	28.3	31.5	70	101
(mozzarella cheese, skim)	288	3.2	27.6	18.0	56	66
Egg beaters	51	2.0	10.3	0	0	0
(no alternate identified)						
Egg beaters with cheese	130	3.1	14.1	6.0	42	5
(egg beaters)	51	2.0	10.3	0	0	0
Egg salad	369	1.8	10.0	35.7	87	455
(potato salad)	162	12.7	3.1	9.3	52	77
Egg whites	51	0	13.7	0	0	0
(no alternate identified)						
Egg yolk fresh	399	0	19.9	33.2	75	1416
(egg whites)	51	0	13.7	0	0	0
Eggnog	153	15.3	4.3	8.5	50	67
(chocolate milk, 1% low fat)	71	11.8	3.6	1.1	14	3
Eggs, fried	225	1.54	15.3	17.0	68	519
(egg beaters)	51	2.0	10.3	0	0	0
Eggs, hard boiled	170	1.1	13.6	11.3	60	481
(egg beaters)	51	2.0	10.3	0	0	0
Eggs, poached	170	1.1	13.6	11.3	60	479
(egg beaters)	51	2.0	10.3	0	0	0
Eggs, scrambled	185	1.9	13.0	13.0	63	398
(egg beaters)	51	2.0	10.3	0	0	0
Eggs, whole, raw	170	1.1	13.6	11.3	60	481
(egg beaters)	51	2.0	10.3	0	0	0

( ) indicates possible substitute foods that are lower in calories and/or fat.

Serving size--4 ounces:	Calories kcal	Carbo grams	Prot grams	Fat grams	Fat % of kcal	Chol mg
Evaporated skim milk	88	12.8	8.5	0.2	2	4
(milk, skim)	40	5.4	3.9	0.2	4	2
Evaporated whole milk	152	11.3	7.7	8.6	51	33
(evaporated skim milk)	88	12.8	8.5	0.2	2	4
Fat-free cheddar cheese	160	4.0	32.0	0	0	12
(cottage cheese, 1% low fat)	82	3.1	14.1	1.1	12	5
Fat-free swiss cheese	160	4.0	32.0	0	0	12
(cottage cheese, 1% low fat)	82	3.1	14.1	1.1	12	5
Feta cheese	299	4.6	16.1	24.2	73	101
(ricotta cheese, part skim)	156	5.8	12.9	9.0	52	35
Fontina cheese	441	1.7	29.0	35.3	72	132
(mozzarella cheese, skim)	288	3.2	27.6	18.0	56	66
Frozen dessert topping	361	26.1	1.5	28.7	72	0
(dessert topping, ready to eat)	214	18.7	4.1	14.1	59	11
Frozen yogurt, nonfat	95	21.0	4.0	0	0	0
(yogurt, plain nonfat)	56	8.1	6.0	0	0	0
Frozen yogurt, regular	99	18.0	2.9	1.9	17	7
(frozen yogurt, nonfat)	95	21.0	4.0	0	0	0
Gjetost cheese	528	48.3	10.9	33.5	57	107
(feta cheese)	299	4.6	16.1	24.2	73	101
Goose eggs, whole	210	1.5	15.8	15.1	65	966
(egg beaters)	51	2.0	10.3	0	0	0
Gouda cheese	404	2.5	28.2	31.1	69	129
(mozzarella cheese, skim)	288	3.2	27.6	18.0	56	66
Grated parmesan cheese	517	4.2	47.2	34.0	59	89
(feta cheese)	299	4.6	16.1	24.2	73	101
Gruyere cheese	468	0.5	33.8	36.6	70	125
(mozzarella cheese, skim)	288	3.2	27.6	18.0	56	66
Half and half cream	147	4.9	3.4	13.0	80	42
(milk, skim)	40	5.4	3.9	0.2	4	2
Hard parmesan cheese	445	3.6	40.6	29.3	59	77
(feta cheese)	299	4.6	16.1	24.2	73	101
Heavy whipping cream	391	3.2	2.3	42.0	97	155
(light whipping cream)	331	3.4	2.5	35.0	95	126

( ) indicates possible substitute foods that are lower in calories and/or fat.

Serving size--4 ounces:	Calories kcal	Carbo grams	Prot grams	Fat grams	Fat % of kcal	Chol mg
Ice cream, french vanilla	273	25.4	4.0	18.4	58	69
(ice milk, hard vanilla)	159	25.1	4.4	4.9	28	16
Ice cream, vanilla, 10% fat	229	27.0	4.1	12.2	48	51
(ice milk, hard vanilla)	159	25.1	4.4	4.9	28	16
Ice cream, vanilla, 16% fat	268	24.5	3.2	18.1	61	67
(ice milk, hard vanilla)	159	25.1	4.4	4.9	28	16
Ice milk, hard vanilla	159	25.1	4.4	4.9	28	16
(frozen yogurt, nonfat)	95	21.0	4.0	0	0	0
Ice milk, soft, vanilla	143	24.8	5.2	2.9	18	14
(frozen yogurt, nonfat)	95	21.0	4.0	0	0	0
Imitation milk with vegetable oil	69	7.0	2.0	3.9	51	0
(milk, skim)	40	5.4	3.9	0.2	4	2
Imitation sour cream	236	7.5	2.7	22.1	84	0
(sour half and half)	153	4.9	3.3	13.6	80	44
Light table cream	221	4.2	3.1	21.9	89	75
(half and half cream)	147	4.9	3.4	13.0	80	42
Light whipping cream	331	3.4	2.5	35.0	95	126
(light table cream)	221	4.2	3.1	21.9	89	75
Limburger cheese	371	0.6	22.7	31.0	75	102
(mozzarella cheese, skim)	288	3.2	27.6	18.0	56	66
Margarine	815	1.0	1.0	91.3	99	0
(promise ultra fat-free margarine)	37	0	0	0	0	0
Medium 25% fat cream	277	4.0	2.8	28.3	92	99
(light table cream)	221	4.2	3.1	21.9	89	75
Milk, whole, 3.3% fat	69	5.3	3.7	3.7	48	15
(milk, skim)	40	5.4	3.9	0.2	4	2
Milk, 1% low fat	48	5.4	3.7	1.2	23	5
(milk, skim)	40	5.4	3.9	0.2	4	2
Milk, 1/2% low fat	43	5.4	3.7	0.8	17	3
(milk, skim)	40	5.4	3.9	0.2	4	2
Milk, 2% low fat	57	5.4	3.7	2.2	35	9
(milk, skim)	40	5.4	3.9	0.2	4	2
Milk, goat, whole	78	5.0	4.1	4.6	53	13
(milk, skim)	40	5.4	3.9	0.2	4	2

( ) indicates possible substitute foods that are lower in calories and/or fat.

Serving size--4 ounces:	Calories kcal	Carbo grams	Prot grams	Fat grams	Fat % of kcal	Chol mg
Milk, reindeer	265	4.6	12.2	22.2	75	16
(milk, skim)	40	5.4	3.9	0.2	4	2
Milk shake, chocolate	135	23.9	3.4	3.1	21	12
(chocolate milk, 1% low fat)	71	11.8	3.6	1.1	14	3
Milk shake, vanilla	127	20.2	4.4	3.4	24	13
(chocolate milk, 1% low fat)	71	11.8	3.6	1.1	14	3
Milk, sheep, whole	122	6.1	6.8	7.9	58	31
(milk, skim)	40	5.4	3.9	0.2	4	2
Milk, skim	40	5.4	3.9	0.2	4	2
(water)	0	0	0	0	0	0
Milk, whole, 3.7% fat	73	5.2	3.7	4.2	52	16
(milk, skim)	40	5.4	3.9	0.2	4	2
Monterey cheese	423	0.8	27.8	34.4	73	101
(mozzarella cheese, skim)	288	3.2	27.6	18.0	56	66
Mozzarella cheese, part skim	318	3.5	31.2	19.4	55	61
(mozzarella cheese, skim)	288	3.2	27.6	18.0	56	66
Mozzarella cheese, regular	319	2.5	22.0	24.5	69	89
(mozzarella cheese, skim)	288	3.2	27.6	18.0	56	66
Mozzarella cheese, skim	288	3.2	27.6	18.0	56	66
(ricotta cheese, part skim)	156	5.8	12.9	9.0	52	35
Muenster cheese	417	1.2	26.5	34.0	73	108
(mozzarella cheese, skim)	288	3.2	27.6	18.0	56	66
Neufchatel cheese	295	3.3	11.3	26.5	81	86
(ricotta cheese, part skim)	156	5.8	12.9	9.0	52	35
Omelet, cheese	223	2.2	13.9	17.5	71	373
(egg beaters with cheese)	130	3.1	14.1	6.0	42	5
Omelet, cheese&bacon&mushroom	245	2.3	14.7	19.4	71	315
(egg beaters with cheese)	130	3.1	14.1	6.0	42	5
Omelet, cheese and bacon	256	2.0	15.5	20.4	72	352
(egg beaters with cheese)	130	3.1	14.1	6.0	42	5
Omelet, cheese and tomato	183	2.5	11.3	13.9	68	350
(egg beaters with cheese)	130	3.1	14.1	6.0	42	5
Philly light neufchatel cheese	320	4.0	12.0	28.0	79	100
(cream cheese, philly light soft)	240	8.1	12.0	20.0	75	40

( ) indicates possible substitute foods that are lower in calories and/or fat.

Serving size--4 ounces:	Calories kcal	Carbo grams	Prot grams	Fat grams	Fat % of kcal	Chol mg
Pimento cheese	425	1.9	25.1	35.4	75	107
(mozzarella cheese, skim)	288	3.2	27.6	18.0	56	66
Port du salut cheese	399	0.7	27.0	32.0	72	139
(mozzarella cheese, skim)	288	3.2	27.6	18.0	56	66
Pressurized dessert topping	299	18.3	1.1	25.3	76	0
(dessert topping, ready to eat)	214	18.7	4.1	14.1	59	11
Pressurized whipped cream	291	14.2	3.6	25.2	78	86
(dessert topping, ready to eat)	214	18.7	4.1	14.1	59	11
Provolone cheese	398	2.4	29.0	30.2	68	78
(mozzarella cheese, skim)	288	3.2	27.6	18.0	56	66
Quail eggs, whole	179	0.5	14.7	12.6	63	957
(egg beaters)	51	2.0	10.3	0	0	0
Quiche lorraine	378	9.4	13.5	31.9	76	187
(egg beaters with cheese)	130	3.1	14.1	6.0	42	5
Ricotta cheese, part skim	156	5.8	12.9	9.0	52	35
(cottage cheese, 1% low fat)	82	3.1	14.1	1.1	12	5
Ricotta cheese, regular	197	3.4	12.8	14.7	67	57
(ricotta cheese, part skim)	156	5.8	12.9	9.0	52	35
Romano cheese	439	4.1	36.1	30.5	63	118
(feta cheese)	299	4.6	16.1	24.2	73	101
Roquefort cheese	418	2.3	24.4	34.7	75	102
(feta cheese)	299	4.6	16.1	24.2	73	101
Sherbert	159	34.5	1.2	2.3	13	8
(frozen yogurt, nonfat)	95	21.0	4.0	0	0	0
Sour cream	243	4.9	3.6	23.8	88	50
(sour half and half)	153	4.9	3.3	13.6	80	44
Sour cream & onion dip (chip dip)	248	9.5	4.4	22.1	80	46
(mexican salsa)	25	5.6	1.1	0.2	7	0
Sour half and half	153	4.9	3.3	13.6	80	44
(yogurt, skim, 12g protein/8oz)	64	8.7	6.5	0.2	3	2
Sweet condensed milk	364	61.7	9.0	9.9	24	38
(evaporated skim milk)	88	12.8	8.5	0.2	2	4
Swiss cheese	426	3.9	32.2	31.1	66	104
(feta cheese)	299	4.6	16.1	24.2	73	101

( ) indicates possible substitute foods that are lower in calories and/or fat.

Serving size--4 ounces:	Calories kcal	Carbo grams	Prot grams	Fat grams	Fat % of kcal	Chol mg
Turkey eggs, whole	194	1.2	15.5	13.5	63	1058
(egg beaters)	51	2.0	10.3	0	0	0
Western omelet	183	2.8	11.9	13.5	66	306
(egg beaters with cheese)	130	3.1	14.1	6.0	42	5
Yogurt, plain, 8g protein/8oz	69	5.3	4.0	3.7	48	14
(yogurt, skim, 12g protein/8oz)	64	8.7	6.5	0.2	3	2
Yogurt, plain nonfat	56	8.1	6.0	0	0	0
(no alternate identified)						
Yogurt, skim, 12g protein/8oz	64	8.7	6.5	0.2	3	2
(yogurt, plain nonfat)	56	8.1	6.0	0	0	0
Yogurt w/fruit, low fat	116	21.5	5.0	1.2	9	5
(yogurt, skim, 12g protein/8oz)	64	8.7	6.5	0.2	3	2
Yogurt w/fruit, nonfat	100	20.6	4.6	0	0	0
(yogurt, plain nonfat)	56	8.1	6.0	0	0	0

( ) indicates possible substitute foods that are lower in calories and/or fat.

FRUIT AND JUICE

The serving size for this category is 4 ounces. Please note that for canned fruit the weight, and therefore the nutritional values, include the liquid used in canning.

Weights and Measures

1. One-half cup of juice weighs approximately four ounces.
2. A small apple or orange (2 1/2" diameter) weighs approximately four ounces.
3. Three-quarters cup of grapes weighs approximately four ounces.
4. Three-quarters cup of strawberries weighs approximately four ounces.

Fruit

Serving size--4 ounces:	Calories kcal	Carbo grams	Prot grams	Fat grams	Fat % of kcal	Chol mg
Acerola, fresh	36	8.7	0.5	0.3	7	0
(no alternate identified)						
Acerola juice, fresh	24	5.4	0.5	0.3	11	0
(no alternate identified)						
Apple cider	48	11.7	0.1	0.1	2	0
(tomato juice)	19	4.8	0.9	0.1	5	0
Apple, dried	276	74.7	1.0	0.3	1	0
(apple, fresh)	67	17.4	0.2	0.5	7	0
Apple, fresh	67	17.4	0.2	0.5	7	0
(strawberries, fresh)	34	7.9	0.7	0.5	13	0
Apple juice, from concentrate	53	13.0	0.1	0.1	2	0
(tomato juice)	19	4.8	0.9	0.1	5	0
Apple, without skin	65	16.8	0.1	0.3	4	0
(strawberries, fresh)	34	7.9	0.7	0.5	13	0
Applesauce, canned, sweetened	86	22.6	0.2	0.2	2	0
(applesauce, canned, unsweetened)	49	12.8	0.2	0	0	0
Applesauce, canned, unsweetened	49	12.8	0.2	0	0	0
(strawberries, fresh)	34	7.9	0.7	0.5	13	0
Apricot nectar, canned	64	16.3	0.5	0.1	1	0
(orange juice, fresh)	51	11.8	0.8	0.2	4	0

( ) indicates possible substitute foods that are lower in calories and/or fat.

Serving size--4 ounces:	Calories kcal	Carbo grams	Prot grams	Fat grams	Fat % of kcal	Chol mg
Apricots, candied	383	98.1	0.7	0.2	0	0
(apricots, fresh)	54	12.6	1.6	0.5	8	0
Apricots, canned hvysrp w/skin	94	24.4	0.6	0.1	1	0
(apricots, canned w/water wo/skin)	25	6.2	0.8	0	0	0
Apricots, canned w/juice w/skin	54	13.9	0.7	0	0	0
(apricots, canned w/water wo/skin)	25	6.2	0.8	0	0	0
Apricots, canned w/ltsrp w/skin	71	18.7	0.6	0	0	0
(apricots, canned w/water wo/skin)	25	6.2	0.8	0	0	0
Apricots, canned w/water wo/skin	25	6.2	0.8	0	0	0
(no alternate identified)						
Apricots, canned xhvsrp wo/skin	109	28.1	0.6	0	0	0
(apricots, canned w/water wo/skin)	25	6.2	0.8	0	0	0
Apricots, dried	270	70.1	4.1	0.6	2	0
(apricots, fresh)	54	12.6	1.6	0.5	8	0
Apricots, fresh	54	12.6	1.6	0.5	8	0
(strawberries, fresh)	34	7.9	0.7	0.5	13	0
Apricots, frozen, sweetened	111	28.5	0.8	0.1	1	0
(apricots, fresh)	54	12.6	1.6	0.5	8	0
Avocado	183	8.4	2.3	17.4	86	0
(papayas)	44	11.1	0.7	0.1	2	0
Banana, fresh	104	26.5	1.1	0.6	5	0
(apple, fresh)	67	17.4	0.2	0.5	7	0
Blackberries, canned w/heavy syrup	104	26.2	1.5	0.1	1	0
(blackberries, fresh)	59	14.5	0.8	0.5	8	0
Blackberries, fresh	59	14.5	0.8	0.5	8	0
(strawberries, fresh)	34	7.9	0.7	0.5	13	0
Blackberry juice, canned	42	8.8	0.3	0.7	15	0
(tomato juice)	19	4.8	0.9	0.1	5	0
Blueberries, canned w/heavy syrup	100	25.1	0.7	0.3	3	0
(blueberries, fresh)	64	16.0	0.8	0.5	7	0
Blueberries, fresh	64	16.0	0.8	0.5	7	0
(strawberries, fresh)	34	7.9	0.7	0.5	13	0
Blueberries, frozen, sweetened	92	24.8	0.5	0.1	1	0
(blueberries, fresh)	64	16.0	0.8	0.5	7	0

( ) indicates possible substitute foods that are lower in calories and/or fat.

Serving size--4 ounces:	Calories kcal	Carbo grams	Prot grams	Fat grams	Fat % of kcal	Chol mg
Boysenberries, canned w/hvy syrup	100	25.3	1.1	0.1	1	0
(boysenberries, frozen, unsweeten)	57	13.8	1.2	0.3	5	0
Boysenberries, frozen, unsweetened	57	13.8	1.2	0.3	5	0
(strawberries, fresh)	34	7.9	0.7	0.5	13	0
Breadfruit	117	30.7	1.2	0.2	2	0
(papayas)	44	11.1	0.7	0.1	2	0
Candied figs	339	83.6	4.0	0.2	1	0
(figs, fresh)	84	21.8	0.9	0.3	3	0
Candied grapefruit peel	358	91.4	0.5	0.3	1	0
(grapefruit, fresh)	36	9.2	0.7	0.1	2	0
Candied lemon peel	358	91.4	0.5	0.3	1	0
(lemon without peel)	33	10.5	1.2	0.3	8	0
Candied orange peel	358	91.4	0.5	0.3	1	0
(orange, fresh)	53	13.4	1.0	0.1	2	0
Candied pears	344	86.1	1.5	0.7	2	0
(pears, fresh)	67	17.1	0.5	0.5	7	0
Candied pineapple	358	90.7	0.9	0.5	1	0
(pineapple, fresh)	56	14.1	0.5	0.5	8	0
Cantaloupe melon	40	9.5	1.0	0.3	7	0
(casaba melon)	29	7.0	1.0	0.1	3	0
Carambola	37	8.8	0.6	0.3	7	0
(casaba melon)	29	7.0	1.0	0.1	3	0
Carissa	70	15.4	0.6	1.5	19	0
(strawberries, fresh)	34	7.9	0.7	0.5	13	0
Casaba melon	29	7.0	1.0	0.1	3	0
(no alternate identified)						
Cherimoya	107	27.2	1.5	0.5	4	0
(cantaloupe melon)	40	9.5	1.0	0.3	7	0
Cherries, maraschino	132	33.3	0.2	0.2	1	0
(cherries, sweet, canned w/water)	52	13.4	0.9	0.1	2	0
Cherries, sour, canned w/hvy syrup	103	26.4	0.8	0.1	1	0
(cherries, sour, canned w/water)	41	10.1	0.9	0.1	2	0
Cherries, sour, canned w/light syrup	85	21.9	0.8	0.1	1	0
(cherries, sour, canned w/water)	41	10.1	0.9	0.1	2	0

( ) indicates possible substitute foods that are lower in calories and/or fat.

Serving size--4 ounces:	Calories kcal	Carbo grams	Prot grams	Fat grams	Fat % of kcal	Chol mg
Cherries, sour, canned w/water	41	10.1	0.9	0.1	2	0
(apricots, canned w/water wo/skin)	25	6.2	0.8	0	0	0
Cherries, sour, red, fresh	57	13.8	1.1	0.3	5	0
(strawberries, fresh)	34	7.9	0.7	0.5	13	0
Cherries, sweet, canned w/hvy syrup	94	24.2	0.7	0.1	1	0
(cherries, sweet, canned w/water)	52	13.4	0.9	0.1	2	0
Cherries, sweet, canned w/light syrup	76	19.6	0.7	0.1	1	0
(cherries, sweet, canned w/water)	52	13.4	0.9	0.1	2	0
Cherries, sweet, canned w/juice	61	15.6	1.0	0	0	0
(cherries, sweet, canned w/water)	52	13.4	0.9	0.1	2	0
Cherries, sweet, canned w/water	52	13.4	0.9	0.1	2	0
(strawberries, fresh)	34	7.9	0.7	0.5	13	0
Cherries, sweet, fresh	82	18.7	1.4	1.1	12	0
(cherries, sour, red, fresh)	57	13.8	1.1	0.3	5	0
Citron, candied	356	90.9	0.2	0.3	1	0
(apple, fresh)	67	17.4	0.2	0.5	7	0
Coconut meat, raw	401	17.2	3.7	38.0	85	0
(pineapple, fresh)	56	14.1	0.5	0.5	8	0
Coconut milk	261	6.2	2.6	27.0	93	0
(pineapple juice, canned)	64	15.6	0.3	0.1	1	0
Crabapple, raw	86	22.6	0.5	0.3	3	0
(apple, fresh)	67	17.4	0.2	0.5	7	0
Cranberries, raw	56	14.4	0.5	0.2	3	0
(strawberries, fresh)	34	7.9	0.7	0.5	13	0
Cranberry juice cocktail	66	16.9	0	0	0	0
(orange juice, fresh)	51	11.8	0.8	0.2	4	0
Cranberry sauce, canned, sweetened	171	44.1	0.2	0.1	1	0
(cherries, sweet, canned w/water)	52	13.4	0.9	0.1	2	0
Currants, black, raw	71	17.5	1.6	0.5	6	0
(strawberries, fresh)	34	7.9	0.7	0.5	13	0
Currants, red/white, raw	64	15.6	1.6	0.2	3	0
(strawberries, fresh)	34	7.9	0.7	0.5	13	0
Currants, zante, dried	321	84.0	4.6	0.3	1	0
(currants, red/white, raw)	64	15.6	1.6	0.2	3	0

( ) indicates possible substitute foods that are lower in calories and/or fat.

Serving size--4 ounces:	Calories kcal	Carbo grams	Prot grams	Fat grams	Fat % of kcal	Chol mg
Custard-apple	115	28.6	1.9	0.7	5	0
(apple, fresh)	67	17.4	0.2	0.5	7	0
Dates	312	83.3	2.3	0.5	1	0
(figs, fresh)	84	21.8	0.9	0.3	3	0
Dried fruit	276	72.7	2.8	0.6	2	0
(apple, fresh)	67	17.4	0.2	0.5	7	0
Elderberries	83	20.9	0.8	0.6	7	0
(blueberries, fresh)	64	16.0	0.8	0.5	7	0
Figs, canned with heavy syrup	100	26.0	0.5	0.1	1	0
(figs, fresh)	84	21.8	0.9	0.3	3	0
Figs, dried	289	74.1	3.4	1.4	4	0
(figs, fresh)	84	21.8	0.9	0.3	3	0
Figs, fresh	84	21.8	0.9	0.3	3	0
(strawberries, fresh)	34	7.9	0.7	0.5	13	0
Fruit cocktail, canned w/juice	52	13.5	0.6	0	0	0
(fruit cocktail, canned w/water)	36	9.6	0.5	0	0	0
Fruit cocktail, canned w/water	36	9.6	0.5	0	0	0
(apricots, canned w/water wo/skin)	25	6.2	0.8	0	0	0
Fruit cocktail, extra-heavy syrup	100	26.0	0.5	0.1	1	0
(fruit cocktail, canned w/water)	36	9.6	0.5	0	0	0
Fruit cocktail, heavy syrup	83	21.4	0.5	0.1	1	0
(fruit cocktail, canned w/water)	36	9.6	0.5	0	0	0
Fruit cocktail, light syrup	65	16.9	0.5	0.1	1	0
(fruit cocktail, canned w/water)	36	9.6	0.5	0	0	0
Fruit salad, canned, heavy syrup	83	21.7	0.3	0.1	1	0
(fruit salad, canned with water)	34	9.0	0.3	0.1	3	0
Fruit salad, canned, light syrup	66	17.1	0.3	0.1	1	0
(fruit salad, canned with water)	34	9.0	0.3	0.1	3	0
Fruit salad, canned with juice	57	14.7	0.6	0	0	0
(fruit salad, canned with water)	34	9.0	0.3	0.1	3	0
Fruit salad, canned with water	34	9.0	0.3	0.1	3	0
(apricots, canned w/water wo/skin)	25	6.2	0.8	0	0	0
Fruit salad, tropical	98	25.4	0.5	0.2	2	0
(fruit salad, canned with water)	34	9.0	0.3	0.1	3	0

( ) indicates possible substitute foods that are lower in calories and/or fat.

Serving size--4 ounces:	Calories kcal	Carbo grams	Prot grams	Fat grams	Fat % of kcal	Chol mg
Gooseberries, canned w/light syrup	83	21.3	0.7	0.2	2	0
(gooseberries, fresh)	50	11.6	1.0	0.7	13	0
Gooseberries, fresh	50	11.6	1.0	0.7	13	0
(strawberries, fresh)	34	7.9	0.7	0.5	13	0
Grape juice, canned/bottled	69	17.0	0.7	0.1	1	0
(tomato juice)	19	4.8	0.9	0.1	5	0
Grape juice, sweetened	58	14.5	0.2	0.1	2	0
(tomato juice)	19	4.8	0.9	0.1	5	0
Grapefruit, canned w/light syrup	68	17.5	0.7	0.1	1	0
(grapefruit, fresh)	36	9.2	0.7	0.1	2	0
Grapefruit drink, canned	61	15.6	0.1	0	0	0
(grapefruit juice, fresh-squeezed)	44	10.4	0.6	0.1	2	0
Grapefruit, fresh	36	9.2	0.7	0.1	2	0
(casaba melon)	29	7.0	1.0	0.1	3	0
Grapefruit juice, canned, sweetened	52	12.6	0.7	0.1	2	0
(grapefruit juice, fresh-squeezed)	44	10.4	0.6	0.1	2	0
Grapefruit juice, fresh-squeezed	44	10.4	0.6	0.1	2	0
(tomato juice)	19	4.8	0.9	0.1	5	0
Grapes, canned with heavy syrup	83	22.2	0.6	0.1	1	0
(grapes, fresh, american type)	71	19.4	0.7	0.3	4	0
Grapes, fresh, american type	71	19.4	0.7	0.3	4	0
(strawberries, fresh)	34	7.9	0.7	0.5	13	0
Grapes, fresh, european type	81	20.2	0.8	0.7	8	0
(grapes, fresh, american type)	71	19.4	0.7	0.3	4	0
Ground cherries, raw	60	12.7	2.2	0.8	12	0
(cherries, sour, canned w/water)	41	10.1	0.9	0.1	2	0
Guava sauce	41	10.8	0.3	0.1	2	0
(lemon juice, fresh)	28	9.8	0.5	0	0	0
Guavas, common	58	13.5	0.9	0.7	11	0
(cantaloupe melon)	40	9.5	1.0	0.3	7	0
Guavas, strawberry	78	19.7	0.7	0.7	8	0
(guavas, common)	58	13.5	0.9	0.7	11	0
Honeydew melon	40	10.4	0.6	0.1	2	0
(casaba melon)	29	7.0	1.0	0.1	3	0

( ) indicates possible substitute foods that are lower in calories and/or fat.

Serving size--4 ounces:	Calories kcal	Carbo grams	Prot grams	Fat grams	Fat % of kcal	Chol mg
Jackfruit	107	27.2	1.7	0.3	3	0
(apple, fresh)	67	17.4	0.2	0.5	7	0
Java-plum	68	17.7	0.8	0.2	3	0
(apricots, fresh)	54	12.6	1.6	0.5	8	0
Jujube, raw	90	22.9	1.4	0.2	2	0
(apple, fresh)	67	17.4	0.2	0.5	7	0
Kiwifruit, fresh	69	16.9	1.1	0.5	7	0
(apricots, fresh)	54	12.6	1.6	0.5	8	0
Kumquat	71	18.6	1.0	0.1	1	0
(apricots, fresh)	54	12.6	1.6	0.5	8	0
Lemon juice, fresh	28	9.8	0.5	0	0	0
(no alternate identified)						
Lemon, fresh	33	10.5	1.2	0.3	8	0
(casaba melon)	29	7.0	1.0	0.1	3	0
Lemonade	45	11.9	0.1	0	0	0
(tomato juice)	19	4.8	0.9	0.1	5	0
Lime, fresh	34	11.9	0.8	0.2	5	0
(casaba melon)	29	7.0	1.0	0.1	3	0
Lime ices/water	145	37.0	0.5	0	0	0
(lemonade)	45	11.9	0.1	0	0	0
Lime juice, fresh	31	10.2	0.5	0.1	3	0
(lemon juice, fresh)	28	9.8	0.5	0	0	0
Limeade	46	12.5	0	0	0	0
(tomato juice)	19	4.8	0.9	0.1	5	0
Loganberries	62	14.7	1.7	0.3	4	0
(strawberries, fresh)	34	7.9	0.7	0.5	13	0
Loquat	53	13.7	0.5	0.2	3	0
(strawberries, fresh)	34	7.9	0.7	0.5	13	0
Lychee, fresh	75	18.7	0.9	0.5	6	0
(papayas)	44	11.1	0.7	0.1	2	0
Mango	74	19.3	0.6	0.3	4	0
(papayas)	44	11.1	0.7	0.1	2	0
Mulberries	49	11.1	1.6	0.5	9	0
(strawberries, fresh)	34	7.9	0.7	0.5	13	0

( ) indicates possible substitute foods that are lower in calories and/or fat.

Serving size--4 ounces:	Calories kcal	Carbo grams	Prot grams	Fat grams	Fat % of kcal	Chol mg
Nectarine	56	13.4	1.0	0.6	10	0
(strawberries, fresh)	34	7.9	0.7	0.5	13	0
Orange-apricot juice drink	57	14.4	0.3	0.1	2	0
(orange juice, fresh)	51	11.8	0.8	0.2	4	0
Orange, fresh	53	13.4	1.0	0.1	2	0
(grapefruit, fresh)	36	9.2	0.7	0.1	2	0
Orange juice, fresh	51	11.8	0.8	0.2	4	0
(tomato juice)	19	4.8	0.9	0.1	5	0
Orange juice, from concentrate	51	12.2	0.8	0.1	2	0
(tomato juice)	19	4.8	0.9	0.1	5	0
Papaya nectar	65	16.4	0.2	0.1	1	0
(orange juice, fresh)	51	11.8	0.8	0.2	4	0
Papayas	44	11.1	0.7	0.1	2	0
(strawberries, fresh)	34	7.9	0.7	0.5	13	0
Passion fruit	110	26.5	2.5	0.8	7	0
(apple, fresh)	67	17.4	0.2	0.5	7	0
Passion fruit juice	58	15.4	0.5	0	0	0
(orange juice, fresh)	51	11.8	0.8	0.2	4	0
Peach nectar	61	15.8	0.3	0	0	0
(orange juice, fresh)	51	11.8	0.8	0.2	4	0
Peaches, canned, heavy syrup	84	22.6	0.5	0.1	1	0
(peaches, canned with water)	27	6.9	0.5	0.1	3	0
Peaches, canned, light syrup	61	16.4	0.5	0	0	0
(peaches, canned with water)	27	6.9	0.5	0.1	3	0
Peaches, canned with juice	50	13.2	0.7	0	0	0
(peaches, canned with water)	27	6.9	0.5	0.1	3	0
Peaches, canned with water	27	6.9	0.5	0.1	3	0
(apricots, canned w/water wo/skin)	25	6.2	0.8	0	0	0
Peaches, dried	271	69.5	4.1	0.9	3	0
(peaches, fresh)	49	12.6	0.8	0.1	2	0
Peaches, fresh	49	12.6	0.8	0.1	2	0
(strawberries, fresh)	34	7.9	0.7	0.5	13	0
Peaches, frozen, sweetened	107	27.2	0.7	0.1	1	0
(peaches, fresh)	49	12.6	0.8	0.1	2	0

( ) indicates possible substitute foods that are lower in calories and/or fat.

Serving size--4 ounces:	Calories kcal	Carbo grams	Prot grams	Fat grams	Fat % of kcal	Chol mg
Peaches, spiced, heavy syrup	85	22.8	0.5	0.1	1	0
(peaches, fresh)	49	12.6	0.8	0.1	2	0
Pear nectar	68	17.9	0.1	0	0	0
(orange juice, fresh)	51	11.8	0.8	0.2	4	0
Pears, canned, heavy syrup	84	21.8	0.2	0.1	1	0
(pears, canned with water)	33	8.8	0.2	0	0	0
Pears, canned, light syrup	65	17.2	0.2	0	0	0
(pears, canned with water)	33	8.8	0.2	0	0	0
Pears, canned with juice	57	14.6	0.3	0.1	2	0
(pears, canned with water)	33	8.8	0.2	0	0	0
Pears, canned with water	33	8.8	0.2	0	0	0
(apricots, canned w/water wo/skin)	25	6.2	0.8	0	0	0
Pears, dried	297	79.0	2.2	0.7	2	0
(pears, fresh)	67	17.1	0.5	0.5	7	0
Pears, fresh	67	17.1	0.5	0.5	7	0
(strawberries, fresh)	34	7.9	0.7	0.5	13	0
Persimmon, japan, dried	311	83.2	1.6	0.7	2	0
(persimmon, japan, raw)	79	21.1	0.7	0.2	2	0
Persimmon, japan, raw	79	21.1	0.7	0.2	2	0
(apple, fresh)	67	17.4	0.2	0.5	7	0
Persimmon, native, raw	144	38.0	0.9	0.5	3	0
(persimmon, japan, raw)	79	21.1	0.7	0.2	2	0
Pineapple-grapefruit juice drink	53	13.1	0.2	0.1	2	0
(grapefruit juice, fresh-squeezed)	44	10.4	0.6	0.1	2	0
Pineapple-orange juice drink	57	13.4	1.5	0	0	0
(orange juice, fresh)	51	11.8	0.8	0.2	4	0
Pineapple, canned, heavy syrup	88	22.9	0.3	0.1	1	0
(pineapple, canned with juice)	68	17.8	0.5	0.1	1	0
Pineapple, canned w/light syrup	59	15.2	0.5	0.1	2	0
(strawberries, fresh)	34	7.9	0.7	0.5	13	0
Pineapple, canned with juice	68	17.8	0.5	0.1	1	0
(pineapple, fresh)	56	14.1	0.5	0.5	8	0
Pineapple, fresh	56	14.1	0.5	0.5	8	0
(strawberries, fresh)	34	7.9	0.7	0.5	13	0

( ) indicates possible substitute foods that are lower in calories and/or fat.

Serving size--4 ounces:	Calories kcal	Carbo grams	Prot grams	Fat grams	Fat % of kcal	Chol mg
Pineapple, frozen, sweetened	96	25.2	0.5	0.1	1	0
(pineapple, fresh)	56	14.1	0.5	0.5	8	0
Pineapple juice, canned	64	15.6	0.3	0.1	1	0
(orange juice, fresh)	51	11.8	0.8	0.2	4	0
Plantain	138	36.2	1.5	0.5	3	0
(papayas)	44	11.1	0.7	0.1	2	0
Plums, canned, heavy syrup	101	26.3	0.5	0.1	1	0
(plums, canned with juice)	66	17.1	0.6	0	0	0
Plums, canned with juice	66	17.1	0.6	0	0	0
(strawberries, fresh)	34	7.9	0.7	0.5	13	0
Plums, canned with light syrup	71	18.5	0.5	0.1	1	0
(plums, canned with juice)	66	17.1	0.6	0	0	0
Plums, fresh	62	14.7	0.9	0.7	10	0
(strawberries, fresh)	34	7.9	0.7	0.5	13	0
Pomegranates	77	19.5	1.0	0.3	4	0
(apple, fresh)	67	17.4	0.2	0.5	7	0
Prickly pears	46	10.9	0.8	0.6	12	0
(strawberries, fresh)	34	7.9	0.7	0.5	13	0
Prune juice, canned	81	19.7	0.7	0	0	0
(orange juice, fresh)	51	11.8	0.8	0.2	4	0
Prune whip	177	41.8	5.0	0.2	1	0
(plums, fresh)	62	14.7	0.9	0.7	10	0
Prunes, canned, heavy syrup	119	31.5	1.0	0.2	2	0
(plums, fresh)	62	14.7	0.9	0.7	10	0
Prunes, dried	271	71.1	2.9	0.6	2	0
(plums, fresh)	62	14.7	0.9	0.7	10	0
Quinces	65	17.4	0.5	0.1	1	0
(casaba melon)	29	7.0	1.0	0.1	3	0
Raisins	340	89.7	3.6	0.6	2	0
(grapes, fresh, american type)	71	19.4	0.7	0.3	4	0
Raspberries, canned, heavy syrup	103	26.5	0.9	0.1	1	0
(raspberries, fresh)	56	13.2	1.0	0.6	10	0
Raspberries, fresh	56	13.2	1.0	0.6	10	0
(strawberries, fresh)	34	7.9	0.7	0.5	13	0

( ) indicates possible substitute foods that are lower in calories and/or fat.

Serving size--4 ounces:	Calories kcal	Carbo grams	Prot grams	Fat grams	Fat % of kcal	Chol mg
Raspberries, frozen, sweetened	117	29.7	0.8	0.2	2	0
(raspberries, fresh)	56	13.2	1.0	0.6	10	0
Red bananas	102	26.5	1.4	0.2	2	0
(apple, fresh)	67	17.4	0.2	0.5	7	0
Roselle	56	12.8	1.1	0.7	11	0
(strawberries, fresh)	34	7.9	0.7	0.5	13	0
Sapodilla	94	22.7	0.5	1.2	11	0
(apple, fresh)	67	17.4	0.2	0.5	7	0
Sapotes	152	38.3	2.4	0.7	4	0
(apple, fresh)	67	17.4	0.2	0.5	7	0
Soursop	75	19.1	1.1	0.3	4	0
(apple, fresh)	67	17.4	0.2	0.5	7	0
Strawberries, fresh	34	7.9	0.7	0.5	13	0
(casaba melon)	29	7.0	1.0	0.1	3	0
Strawberries, frozen, sweetened	88	23.8	0.6	0.1	1	0
(strawberries, fresh)	34	7.9	0.7	0.5	13	0
Sugar-apple	107	26.8	2.4	0.3	3	0
(apple, fresh)	67	17.4	0.2	0.5	7	0
Tamarinds	271	70.9	3.2	0.7	2	0
(apple, fresh)	67	17.4	0.2	0.5	7	0
Tangerine juice, fresh	49	11.5	0.6	0.2	4	0
(tomato juice)	19	4.8	0.9	0.1	5	0
Tangerines, canned with juice	42	10.9	0.7	0	0	0
(apricots, canned w/water wo/skin)	25	6.2	0.8	0	0	0
Tangerines, fresh	50	12.7	0.7	0.2	4	0
(strawberries, fresh)	34	7.9	0.7	0.5	13	0
Tangerines, light syrup	69	18.4	0.5	0.1	1	0
(tangerines, canned with juice)	42	10.9	0.7	0	0	0
Tangelo juice	46	11.0	0.6	0.1	2	0
(tomato juice)	19	4.8	0.9	0.1	5	0
Tomato juice	19	4.8	0.9	0.1	5	0
(water)	0	0	0	0	0	0
Watermelon, fresh	36	8.2	0.7	0.5	12	0
(casaba melon)	29	7.0	1.0	0.1	3	0

( ) indicates possible substitute foods that are lower in calories and/or fat.

MISCELLANEOUS FOODS

This category is comprised of foods that are not easily classified as belonging to one of the other categories. It includes ethnic foods and combination foods (i.e., foods that have major characteristics of more than one food category, like beef stew, chicken fried rice, crab meat quiche, etc.). The serving size for this category is 4 ounces, a portion corresponding roughly to a side-dish serving. Some of the foods in this category are typically served as entrees, in which case the appropriate serving would be larger, perhaps 8 ounces.

Weights and Measures

1. A three-egg omelet weighs approximately eight ounces.
2. One-half cup of chicken chow mein weighs approximately four ounces.
3. One-half cup of chili con carne weighs approximately four ounces.
4. One-half cup of rice pudding with raisins weighs approximately five ounces.
5. One-half cup of Spanish rice weighs approximately four ounces.

Serving size--4 ounces:	Calories kcal	Carbo grams	Prot grams	Fat grams	Fat % of kcal	Chol mg
Au gratin potatoes	150	12.8	5.8	8.6	52	26
(scalloped potatoes)	98	12.2	3.3	4.2	39	14
Bagel with cream cheese	332	43.4	11.1	13.4	36	37
(bagel, plain)	312	60.5	11.9	1.8	5	0
Bean and cheese burrito	230	33.5	9.2	7.1	28	17
(taco salad with chili)	126	11.6	7.6	5.7	41	2
Bean burrito	213	31.9	7.4	6.5	27	8
(baked beans (without pork) canned)	105	23.2	5.4	0.5	4	0
Beans and franks, canned	163	14.3	8.6	8.1	45	15
(baked beans (without pork) canned)	105	23.2	5.4	0.5	4	0
Beef and bean burrito	249	32.4	11.0	8.7	31	24
(bean burrito)	213	31.9	7.4	6.5	27	8
Beef and rice casserole	146	16.8	7.5	5.1	31	23
(beef and vegetable stew, canned)	90	8.1	6.6	3.5	35	16

( ) indicates possible substitute foods that are lower in calories and/or fat.

Serving size--4 ounces:	Calories kcal	Carbo grams	Prot grams	Fat grams	Fat % of kcal	Chol mg
Beef and vegetable stew	101	7.0	7.3	4.9	44	29
(beef and vegetable stew, canned)	90	8.1	6.6	3.5	35	16
Beef and vegetable stew, canned	90	8.1	6.6	3.5	35	16
(vegetable chunky ready serve soup)	58	9.0	1.7	1.7	26	0
Beef burrito w/cheese	238	22.8	12.9	10.3	39	35
(bean burrito)	213	31.9	7.4	6.5	27	8
Beef chimichanga	277	27.9	12.8	12.8	42	6
(taco salad with chili)	126	11.6	7.6	5.7	41	2
Beef enchiladas	357	40.9	13.2	15.2	38	41
(bean burrito)	213	31.9	7.4	6.5	27	8
Beef fried rice	168	19.4	6.0	7.3	39	61
(white rice, cooked)	124	27.4	2.3	0.1	1	0
Beef ravioli	117	12.9	5.6	4.6	35	10
(spaghetti with tomato sauce)	99	20.8	3.2	0.3	3	0
Beef stroganoff	204	14.1	10.8	11.5	51	40
(beef and vegetable stew, canned)	90	8.1	6.6	3.5	35	16
Beef teriyaki	299	5.2	20.4	20.8	63	71
(beef, flank steak, lean, cooked)	235	0	30.7	11.5	44	76
Biscuit w/ egg, cheese and bacon	375	26.3	12.8	24.7	59	205
(biscuit with egg)	263	20.2	9.3	16.8	57	194
Biscuit with egg	263	20.2	9.3	16.8	57	194
(egg beaters)	51	2.0	10.3	0	0	0
Biscuit with egg and ham	261	17.9	12.0	16.0	55	177
(egg beaters with cheese)	130	3.1	14.1	6.0	42	5
Biscuit with egg and sausage	366	26.0	12.0	24.4	60	191
(biscuit with egg and ham)	261	17.9	12.0	16.0	55	177
Biscuit with sausage	443	36.6	11.1	29.0	59	32
(biscuits)	401	50.5	7.9	18.5	42	3
Bread pudding/raisin	212	32.2	6.4	6.9	29	77
(low-calorie pudding, prepared)	65	11.1	3.7	0	0	0
Burrito w/ beans, cheese and beef	185	22.1	8.2	7.4	36	69
(taco salad with chili)	126	11.6	7.6	5.7	41	2
Cheese and bacon omelet	256	2.0	15.5	20.4	72	352
(egg beaters with cheese)	130	3.1	14.1	6.0	42	5

( ) indicates possible substitute foods that are lower in calories and/or fat.

Serving size--4 ounces:	Calories kcal	Carbo grams	Prot grams	Fat grams	Fat % of kcal	Chol mg
Cheese and beef enchiladas	191	18.0	7.0	10.4	49	24
(taco salad with chili)	126	11.6	7.6	5.7	41	2
Cheese and sausage pizza	320	31.1	14.6	15.1	42	33
(pizza with mushrooms)	238	28.8	12.2	8.3	31	18
Cheese and tomato omelet	183	2.5	11.3	13.9	68	350
(egg beaters with cheese)	130	3.1	14.1	6.0	42	5
Cheese fondue	301	11.3	16.8	20.8	62	254
(cheese soup with milk)	104	7.4	4.3	6.6	56	22
Cheese omelet	223	2.2	13.9	17.5	71	373
(egg beaters with cheese)	130	3.1	14.1	6.0	42	5
Cheese ravioli	118	16.8	4.0	4.0	31	3
(spaghetti with tomato sauce)	99	20.8	3.2	0.3	3	0
Cheese souffle	247	7.0	11.2	19.4	71	210
(low-calorie pudding, prepared)	64	11.2	3.8	0	0	0
Chicken a la king	217	5.7	12.7	15.9	66	86
(chicken breast, meat only, roasted)	187	0	35.2	4.1	20	96
Chicken and rice casserole	129	17.2	9.1	2.4	17	23
(chicken chow mein, canned)	43	8.1	2.9	0.1	2	3
Chicken chow mein, canned	43	8.1	2.9	0.1	2	3
(chicken gumbo soup)	26	3.8	1.2	0.7	24	1.7
Chicken chow mein, homemade	116	4.5	14.1	4.5	35	35
(chicken chow mein, canned)	43	8.1	2.9	0.1	2	3
Chicken cordon bleu	217	3.9	27.1	9.6	40	88
(chicken breast, meat only, roasted)	187	0	35.2	4.1	20	96
Chicken dijon	219	1.5	29.3	10.2	42	81
(chicken breast, meat only, roasted)	187	0	35.2	4.1	20	96
Chicken enchiladas	339	41.4	14.9	12.2	32	41
(bean burrito)	213	31.9	7.4	6.5	27	8
Chicken fricassee	183	3.6	17.4	10.5	52	45
(chicken chow mein, canned)	43	8.1	2.9	0.1	2	3
Chicken fried rice	158	19.6	6.1	5.9	34	61
(white rice, cooked)	124	27.4	2.3	0.1	1	0
Chicken kiev	388	18.8	19.1	26.0	60	193
(chicken breast, meat only, roasted)	187	0	35.2	4.1	20	96

( ) indicates possible substitute foods that are lower in calories and/or fat.

Serving size--4 ounces:	Calories kcal	Carbo grams	Prot grams	Fat grams	Fat % of kcal	Chol mg
Chicken liver pate	228	7.4	15.2	14.9	59	443
(chicken spread, canned)	218	6.1	17.5	13.3	55	59
Chicken parmesan	232	8.4	20.4	12.8	50	66
(chicken breast, meat only, roasted)	187	0	35.2	4.1	20	96
Chicken potpie, frozen, cooked	248	25.2	7.6	13.0	47	15
(chicken chow mein, canned)	43	8.1	2.9	0.1	2	3
Chicken potpie, homemade	266	20.8	11.5	15.3	52	35
(chicken chow mein, canned)	43	8.1	2.9	0.1	2	3
Chile con carne with beans	151	13.8	8.5	6.9	41	19
(baked beans (without pork) canned)	105	23.2	5.4	0.5	4	0
Chile con carne without beans	227	6.6	11.7	16.8	67	29
(chili con carne with beans)	151	13.8	8.5	6.9	41	19
Chile con queso	277	3.2	16.8	21.9	71	70
(refried beans)	238	34.4	10.4	6.9	26	6
Chinese fried rice	163	19.4	4.8	7.1	39	59
(white rice, cooked)	124	27.4	2.3	0.1	1	0
Chop suey with meat, canned	70	4.8	5.0	3.6	46	14
(chicken chow mein, canned)	43	8.1	2.9	0.1	2	3
Chop suey with meat, homemade	136	5.8	11.8	7.7	51	45
(chicken chow mein, homemade)	116	4.5	14.1	4.5	35	35
Corn dog	298	36.2	10.9	12.2	37	51
(turkey sandwich)	201	23.8	18.1	2.3	11	27
Corned beef hash, canned	205	12.1	10.0	12.8	56	37
(beef fried rice)	168	19.4	6.0	7.3	39	61
Crab imperial	167	4.4	16.6	8.6	46	159
(steamed crab)	105	0.6	19.6	2.2	19	113
Crab meat quiche	280	9.0	10.2	22.7	73	191
(steamed crab)	105	0.6	19.6	2.2	19	113
Croissant w/egg, sausage & cheese	371	17.5	14.4	27.0	65	153
(croissant with egg and cheese)	329	21.7	11.5	22.0	60	193
Croissant with egg and cheese	329	21.7	11.5	22.0	60	193
(english muffin, plain)	266	52.1	8.7	2.0	7	0
Curried rice	204	28.1	4.2	9.0	40	7
(white rice, cooked)	124	27.4	2.3	0.1	1	0

( ) indicates possible substitute foods that are lower in calories and/or fat.

Serving size--4 ounces:	Calories kcal	Carbo grams	Prot grams	Fat grams	Fat % of kcal	Chol mg
Deluxe potato skins, baked	295	30.6	12.6	13.8	42	34
(potatoes, baked, with skin)	124	28.6	2.6	0.1	1	0
Deviled crab	213	15.1	12.9	10.7	45	116
(steamed crab)	105	0.6	19.6	2.2	19	113
Egg rolls	220	21.1	5.0	13.3	54	4
(chinese fried rice)	163	19.4	4.8	7.1	39	59
English muffin, cheese and sausage	335	28.8	14.9	21.2	57	188
(english muffin,egg cheese&can bcn)	297	24.4	15.4	15.3	46	181
English muffin,egg cheese&can bcn	297	24.4	15.4	15.3	46	181
(english muffin, plain)	266	52.1	8.7	2.0	7	0
English muffin,egg cheese sausage	335	20.5	14.9	21.2	57	188
(english muffin,egg cheese&can bcn)	297	24.4	15.4	15.3	46	181
Fettucini alfredo	279	16.1	6.2	21.2	68	68
(spaghetti with tomato sauce)	99	20.8	3.2	0.3	3	0
Fish, american shad, creole	172	1.8	17.0	9.9	52	50
(shrimp creole)	79	5.3	12.7	0.7	8	94
Fish, black bass, baked stuffed	294	12.9	18.4	17.9	55	52
(bluefish, baked/broiled)	180	0	29.7	5.9	29	79
French toast	269	40.5	10.4	6.8	23	250
(english muffin, plain)	243	54.7	8.5	1.7	6	0
Frozen beef potpie	218	20.4	8.3	11.2	46	20
(beef and vegetable stew, canned)	90	8.1	6.6	3.5	35	16
Gnocchi (in tomato sauce)	126	26.9	3.6	0.6	4	1
(spaghetti with tomato sauce)	99	20.8	3.2	0.3	3	0
Goose liver pate	524	5.3	12.9	49.7	85	170
(chicken spread, canned)	218	6.1	17.5	13.3	55	59
Green bean casserole	83	10.8	2.2	4.0	43	0
(green beans (string beans), canned)	17	4.0	0.9	0.1	5	0
Guacamole dip	189	7.1	2.4	18.6	89	0
(mexican salsa)	25	5.6	1.1	0.2	7	0
Homemade beef potpie, baked	279	21.3	11.5	16.4	53	24
(beef and vegetable stew, canned)	90	8.1	6.6	3.5	35	16
Lasagne, prepared	204	23.1	10.5	7.6	34	28
(spaghetti with tomato sauce)	99	20.8	3.2	0.3	3	0

( ) indicates possible substitute foods that are lower in calories and/or fat.

Serving size--4 ounces:	Calories kcal	Carbo grams	Prot grams	Fat grams	Fat % of kcal	Chol mg
Macaroni & cheese, canned	108	12.1	4.4	4.5	37	11
(spaghetti with tomato sauce)	99	20.8	3.2	0.3	3	0
Macaroni & cheese, homemade	244	22.8	9.5	12.6	46	39
(spaghetti with tomato sauce)	99	20.8	3.2	0.3	3	0
Manicotti, prepared	152	16.6	7.6	6.1	36	23
(spaghetti with tomato sauce)	99	20.8	3.2	0.3	3	0
Mashed potatoes, w/milk & marg	120	18.9	2.2	4.8	36	2
(potatoes, baked, without skin)	105	24.5	2.3	0.1	1	0
Meatloaf	303	6.1	23.8	19.6	58	129
(chicken breast, meat only, roasted)	187	0	35.2	4.1	20	96
Mexican salsa	25	5.6	1.1	0.2	7	0
(no alternate identified)						
Nachos	439	32.4	15.5	29.8	61	50
(bean burrito)	213	31.9	7.4	6.5	27	8
Nachos w/cheese, beef, peppers	253	24.8	8.8	13.6	48	9
(taco salad with chili)	126	11.6	7.6	5.7	41	2
Nachos grande	268	17.8	11.2	17.9	60	37
(bean burrito)	213	31.9	7.4	6.5	27	8
Pasta, spaghetti w/meat balls, canned	117	12.9	5.6	4.6	35	10
(spaghetti with tomato sauce)	99	20.8	3.2	0.3	3	0
Pasta, spaghetti, tomato sauce/cheese	118	16.8	4.0	4.0	31	3
(spaghetti with tomato sauce)	99	20.8	3.2	0.3	3	0
Pasta, spaghetti with meat balls	152	17.7	8.5	5.3	31	34
(spaghetti with tomato sauce)	99	20.8	3.2	0.3	3	0
Pasta with carbonara sauce	442	34.8	20.0	24.0	49	171
(spaghetti with tomato sauce)	99	20.8	3.2	0.3	3	0
Peppers, sweet, stuffed	193	19.1	14.7	6.2	29	43
(sweet pepper, canned)	20	4.4	0.9	0.3	13	0
Plain chinese fried rice	150	21.2	3.4	5.4	32	57
(white rice, cooked)	124	27.4	2.3	0.1	1	0
Pork and beans (baked beans) canned	138	21.5	6.9	2.9	19	5
(navy beans, canned)	76	14.7	6.9	0.8	9	0
Potato skins w/cheese & bacon	336	33.0	14.3	16.4	44	41
(potatoes, baked, with skin)	124	28.6	2.6	0.1	1	0

( ) indicates possible substitute foods that are lower in calories and/or fat.

Serving size--4 ounces:	Calories kcal	Carbo grams	Prot grams	Fat grams	Fat % of kcal	Chol mg
Potato skins w/cheese, baked	288	37.4	11.5	10.7	33	34
(potatoes, baked, with skin)	124	28.6	2.6	0.1	1	0
Quesadillas	443	46.4	17.5	20.5	42	57
(bean burrito)	213	31.9	7.4	6.5	27	8
Quiche lorraine	378	9.4	13.5	31.9	76	187
(egg beaters with cheese)	130	3.1	14.1	6.0	42	5
Refried beans	238	34.5	10.4	6.9	26	6
(pinto beans, canned)	88	16.5	5.2	0.3	3	0
Rice pudding with raisins	166	30.3	4.1	3.5	19	12
(low-calorie pudding, prepared)	65	11.1	3.7	0	0	0
Salmon rice loaf	138	8.3	13.6	5.1	33	24
(spanish rice, cooked)	99	18.8	2.0	1.9	17	0
Scalloped potatoes	98	12.2	3.3	4.2	39	14
(green beans (string beans), canned)	17	4.0	0.9	0.1	5	0
Shrimp creole	79	5.3	12.7	0.7	8	94
(stewed tomatoes, canned)	29	7.4	1.0	0.1	3	0
Shrimp fried rice	145	19.6	4.9	5.0	31	66
(white rice, cooked)	124	27.4	2.3	0.1	1	0
Spanish rice, cooked	99	18.8	2.0	1.9	17	0
(stewed tomatoes, canned)	29	7.4	1.0	0.1	3	0
Spinach souffle	183	2.4	9.2	15.3	75	153
(spinach, canned)	22	3.3	2.4	0.5	20	0
Taco salad	160	13.5	7.6	8.5	48	25
(tossed salad (without dressing))	17	3.2	1.1	0.2	11	0
Taco salad with chili	126	11.6	7.6	5.7	41	2
(tossed salad (without dressing))	17	3.2	1.1	0.2	11	0
Tacos	281	23.0	10.7	17.8	57	32
(bean burrito)	213	31.9	7.4	6.5	27	8
Toast with butter and jelly	393	62.6	8.2	12.1	28	28
(english muffin, plain)	266	52.1	8.7	2.0	7	0
Tostados	281	23.0	10.7	17.8	57	32
(bean burrito)	213	31.9	7.4	6.5	27	8
Tuna noodle casserole	198	19.5	9.5	9.0	41	38
(spaghetti with tomato sauce)	99	20.8	3.2	0.3	3	0

( ) indicates possible substitute foods that are lower in calories and/or fat.

Serving size--4 ounces:	Calories kcal	Carbo grams	Prot grams	Fat grams	Fat % of kcal	Chol mg
Turkey potpie	269	21.0	11.8	15.3	51	35
(turkey, light, meat only, roasted)	178	0	33.9	3.6	18	78
Veal parmesan	346	14.4	15.5	25.3	66	44
(chicken parmesan)	232	8.4	20.4	12.8	50	66
Veal scaloppine	296	5.3	24.9	18.1	55	104
(chicken breast, meat only, roasted)	187	0	35.2	4.1	20	96
Veal scaloppine (with cheese)	316	5.1	26.0	20.1	57	104
(chicken breast, meat only, roasted)	187	0	35.2	4.1	20	96
Western omelet	183	2.8	11.9	13.5	66	306
(egg beaters with cheese)	130	3.1	14.1	6.0	42	5

( ) indicates possible substitute foods that are lower in calories and/or fat.

PASTA, PIZZA AND RICE

The serving size used for pasta, pizza and rice is 4 ounces, an amount roughly equivalent to a side serving or approximately half of a main serving.

Weights and Measures

1. One quarter of a 10" pizza weighs approximately three and one-half ounces.
2. One sixth of a 14" pizza weighs approximately three ounces.
3. One cup of spaghetti with meatballs and tomato sauce weighs approximately nine ounces.
4. One-half cup macaroni and cheese weighs approximately four ounces.
5. One-half cup Spanish rice weighs approximately four ounces.
6. One-half cup cooked rice weighs approximately three ounces.

Serving size--4 ounces:	Calories kcal	Carbo grams	Prot grams	Fat grams	Fat % of kcal	Chol mg
Beef fried rice	168	19.4	6.0	7.3	39	61
(white rice, cooked)	124	27.4	2.3	0.1	1	0
Beef ravioli	117	12.9	5.6	4.6	35	10
(spaghetti with tomato sauce)	99	20.8	3.2	0.3	3	0
Black olive and mushroom pizza	240	27.1	11.5	9.8	37	17
(spaghetti with tomato sauce)	99	20.8	3.2	0.3	3	0
Black olive and pepperoni pizza	286	26.9	13.3	13.9	44	24
(pizza with mushrooms)	238	28.8	12.2	8.3	31	18
Brown rice, cooked	126	26.1	2.9	1.0	7	0
(potatoes, baked, without skin)	105	24.5	2.3	0.1	1	0
Cannelloni w/tomato sauce, cheese	118	16.8	4.0	4.0	31	3
(spaghetti with tomato sauce)	99	20.8	3.2	0.3	3	0
Cheese and sausage pizza	320	31.1	14.6	15.1	42	33
(pizza with mushrooms)	238	28.8	12.2	8.3	31	18
Cheese pizza	268	32.1	13.6	9.4	32	20
(spaghetti with tomato sauce)	99	20.8	3.2	0.3	3	0
Cheese pizza with extra cheese	271	28.5	14.4	11.0	37	28
(pizza with mushrooms)	238	28.8	12.2	8.3	31	18

( ) indicates possible substitute foods that are lower in calories and/or fat.

Serving size--4 ounces:	Calories kcal	Carbo grams	Prot grams	Fat grams	Fat % of kcal	Chol mg
Cheese ravioli	118	16.8	4.0	4.0	31	3
(spaghetti with tomato sauce)	99	20.8	3.2	0.3	3	0
Chicken fried rice	158	19.6	6.1	5.9	34	61
(white rice, cooked)	124	27.4	2.3	0.1	1	0
Combo pizza (4 meat items)	367	23.2	18.1	22.1	54	49
(pizza with mushrooms)	238	28.8	12.2	8.3	31	18
Curried rice	204	28.1	4.2	9.0	40	7
(white rice, cooked)	124	27.4	2.3	0.1	1	0
Egg noodles, cooked	151	28.1	5.4	1.7	10	37
(pasta, cooked tender)	126	26.1	3.9	0.5	4	0
Fettucini alfredo	279	16.1	6.2	21.2	68	68
(spaghetti with tomato sauce)	99	20.8	3.2	0.3	3	0
Gnocchi (in tomato sauce)	126	26.9	3.6	0.6	4	1
(spaghetti with tomato sauce)	99	20.8	3.2	0.3	3	0
Green olive and pepperoni pizza	279	26.8	13.4	13.2	43	24
(pizza with mushrooms)	238	28.8	12.2	8.3	31	18
Instant rice, prepared	111	24.1	2.4	0.2	2	0
(potatoes, baked, without skin)	105	24.5	2.3	0.1	1	0
Lasagne, prepared	204	23.1	10.5	7.6	34	28
(spaghetti with tomato sauce)	99	20.8	3.2	0.3	3	0
Linguini with red clam sauce	119	23.8	4.8	0.5	4	3
(spaghetti with tomato sauce)	99	20.8	3.2	0.3	3	0
Linguini with white clam sauce	174	25.1	5.6	5.4	28	19
(linguini with red clam sauce)	119	23.8	4.8	0.5	4	3
Macaroni & cheese, canned	108	12.1	4.4	4.5	37	11
(spaghetti with tomato sauce)	99	20.8	3.2	0.3	3	0
Macaroni & cheese, homemade	244	22.8	9.5	12.6	46	39
(spaghetti with tomato sauce)	99	20.8	3.2	0.3	3	0
Macaroni and cheese, box, prepared	213	25.1	6.6	9.5	40	26
(spaghetti with tomato sauce)	99	20.8	3.2	0.3	3	0
Macaroni salad/pasta salad	331	19.2	3.1	27.3	74	20
(pasta, cooked tender)	126	26.1	3.9	0.5	4	0
Manicotti, prepared	152	16.6	7.6	6.1	36	23
(spaghetti with tomato sauce)	99	20.8	3.2	0.3	3	0

( ) indicates possible substitute foods that are lower in calories and/or fat.

Serving size--4 ounces:	Calories kcal	Carbo grams	Prot grams	Fat grams	Fat % of kcal	Chol mg
Mushroom and pepperoni pizza	270	27.1	13.4	12.0	40	24
(pizza with mushrooms)	238	28.8	12.2	8.3	31	18
Mushroom and sausage pizza	293	28.6	13.5	13.7	42	30
(pizza with mushrooms)	238	28.8	12.2	8.3	31	18
Pasta, cooked firm	168	34.1	5.7	0.6	3	0
(white rice, cooked)	124	27.4	2.3	0.1	1	0
Pasta, cooked tender	126	26.1	3.9	0.5	4	0
(white rice, cooked)	124	27.4	2.3	0.1	1	0
Pasta with carbonara sauce	442	34.8	20.0	24.0	49	171
(spaghetti with tomato sauce)	99	20.8	3.2	0.3	3	0
Pizza hut cheese pan pizza	273	31.6	16.7	10.0	33	19
(spaghetti with tomato sauce)	99	20.8	3.2	0.3	3	0
Pizza hut hand-tossed cheese	265	28.2	17.5	10.2	35	28
(spaghetti with tomato sauce)	99	20.8	3.2	0.3	3	0
Pizza hut hand-tossed pepperoni	290	29.0	16.2	13.4	42	29
(spaghetti with tomato sauce)	99	20.8	3.2	0.3	3	0
Pizza hut hand-tossed supreme	257	23.8	15.2	12.4	43	26
(spaghetti with tomato sauce)	99	20.8	3.2	0.3	3	0
Pizza hut pepperoni pan pizza	291	33.6	15.6	11.9	37	23
(spaghetti with tomato sauce)	99	20.8	3.2	0.3	3	0
Pizza hut supreme pan pizza	262	23.6	14.2	13.4	46	24
(spaghetti with tomato sauce)	99	20.8	3.2	0.3	3	0
Pizza hut thin'n crispy cheese pizza	306	28.5	21.5	13.0	38	25
(spaghetti with tomato sauce)	99	20.8	3.2	0.3	3	0
Pizza hut thin'n crispy pepperoni	324	28.2	20.4	15.6	43	36
(spaghetti with tomato sauce)	99	20.8	3.2	0.3	3	0
Pizza hut thin'n crispy supreme	262	23.5	16.0	12.6	43	24
(spaghetti with tomato sauce)	99	20.8	3.2	0.3	3	0
Pizza with anchovies	257	28.2	14.4	9.6	34	25
(spaghetti with tomato sauce)	99	20.8	3.2	0.3	3	0
Pizza with bacon	308	28.2	15.9	14.6	43	29
(pizza with mushrooms)	238	28.8	12.2	8.3	31	18
Pizza with black olives	259	28.6	12.1	10.9	38	18
(spaghetti with tomato sauce)	99	20.8	3.2	0.3	3	0

( ) indicates possible substitute foods that are lower in calories and/or fat.

Serving size--4 ounces:	Calories kcal	Carbo grams	Prot grams	Fat grams	Fat % of kcal	Chol mg
Pizza with green olives	249	28.3	12.1	9.9	36	18
(spaghetti with tomato sauce)	99	20.8	3.2	0.3	3	0
Pizza with ham	272	28.1	15.2	10.9	36	30
(pizza with mushrooms)	238	28.8	12.2	8.3	31	18
Pizza with mushrooms	238	28.8	12.2	8.3	31	18
(spaghetti with tomato sauce)	99	20.8	3.2	0.3	3	0
Pizza with onions	239	29.1	12.1	8.3	31	18
(spaghetti with tomato sauce)	99	20.8	3.2	0.3	3	0
Pizza with pepperoni	298	28.6	14.6	13.9	42	28
(pizza with mushrooms)	238	28.8	12.2	8.3	31	18
Pizza with peppers	238	28.8	12.0	8.3	31	18
(spaghetti with tomato sauce)	99	20.8	3.2	0.3	3	0
Pizza with sausage and pepperoni	338	28.5	15.3	17.9	48	37
(pizza with mushrooms)	238	28.8	12.2	8.3	31	18
Pizza with sausage, extra cheese	316	28.3	15.1	15.8	45	37
(pizza with mushrooms)	238	28.8	12.2	8.3	31	18
Plain chinese fried rice	150	21.2	3.4	5.4	32	57
(white rice, cooked)	124	27.4	2.3	0.1	1	0
Pork fried rice	163	19.4	4.8	7.1	39	59
(white rice, cooked)	124	27.4	2.3	0.1	1	0
Rice pudding with raisins	166	30.3	4.1	3.5	19	12
(white rice, cooked)	124	27.4	2.3	0.1	1	0
Rigatoni w/tomato sauce & cheese	118	16.8	4.0	4.0	31	3
(spaghetti with tomato sauce)	99	20.8	3.2	0.3	3	0
Shrimp fried rice	145	19.6	4.9	5.0	31	66
(white rice, cooked)	124	27.4	2.3	0.1	1	0
Spaghetti w/tomato sauce & cheese	118	16.8	4.0	4.0	31	3
(spaghetti with tomato sauce)	99	20.8	3.2	0.3	3	0
Spaghetti with meat balls	152	17.7	8.5	5.3	31	34
(spaghetti with tomato sauce)	99	20.8	3.2	0.3	3	0
Spaghetti with meat balls, canned	117	12.9	5.6	4.6	35	10
(spaghetti with tomato sauce)	99	20.8	3.2	0.3	3	0
Spaghetti with meat sauce	152	17.7	8.5	5.3	31	34
(spaghetti with tomato sauce)	99	20.8	3.2	0.3	3	0

( ) indicates possible substitute foods that are lower in calories and/or fat.

Serving size--4 ounces:	Calories kcal	Carbo grams	Prot grams	Fat grams	Fat % of kcal	Chol mg
Spaghetti with tomato sauce	99	20.8	3.2	0.3	3	0
(shrimp creole)	79	5.3	12.7	0.7	8	94
Spanish rice, cooked	99	18.8	2.0	1.9	17	0
(stewed tomatoes, canned)	29	7.4	1.0	0.1	3	0
Tortellini with white sauce	183	27.7	5.3	5.4	27	16
(spaghetti with tomato sauce)	99	20.8	3.2	0.3	3	0
White rice, cooked	124	27.4	2.3	0.1	1	0
(potatoes, baked, without skin)	105	24.5	2.3	0.1	1	0
Wild rice, cooked	115	24.2	4.5	0.3	2	0
(potatoes, baked, without skin)	105	24.5	2.3	0.1	1	0
Ziti w/tomato sauce and cheese	118	16.8	4.0	4.0	31	3
(spaghetti with tomato sauce)	99	20.8	3.2	0.3	3	0

( ) indicates possible substitute foods that are lower in calories and/or fat.

POULTRY

The serving size for this category is 8 ounces because poultry is typically served as a main dish. This category contains a broad sampling of different types of poultry. Nutritional information is provided on a variety of cuts and preparation methods to facilitate comparisons and selections. This category also contains some products that are a combination of poultry and other foods, like chicken potpie and chicken enchiladas (although these combination foods also appear in the Miscellaneous Foods category).

Weights and Measures

1. One chicken breast half (from a three-pound chicken) weighs approximately four ounces.
2. One chicken wing (from a three-pound chicken) weighs approximately two ounces.
3. One chicken drumstick (from a three-pound chicken) weighs approximately two ounces
4. One slice of chicken roll weighs approximately one ounce (e.g., a one-pound package of chicken roll cut into sixteen slices).

Serving size--8 ounces:	Calories kcal	Carbo grams	Prot grams	Fat grams	Fat % of kcal	Chol mg
Capon giblets, simmered	372	1.8	59.9	12.2	30	984
(chicken giblets, simmered)	356	2.0	58.5	10.9	28	891
Capon meat with skin, roasted	519	0	65.8	26.3	46	195
(chicken breast, meat only, roasted)	374	0	70.3	8.2	20	193
Chicken a la king	433	11.3	25.4	31.8	66	172
(chicken chow mein, canned)	86	16.1	5.9	0.2	2	7
Chicken and noodles, homemade	347	24.3	21.1	17.5	45	91
(chicken chow mein, canned)	86	16.1	5.9	0.2	2	7
Chicken back meat, fried	653	12.9	68.0	34.7	48	211
(chicken back meat, roasted)	542	0	64.0	29.9	50	204
Chicken back meat, roasted	542	0	64.0	29.9	50	204
(chicken breast, meat only, roasted)	374	0	70.3	8.2	20	193
Chicken back meat, stewed	474	0	57.4	25.4	48	193
(chicken breast, meat only, stewed)	342	0	65.8	6.8	18	175

( ) indicates possible substitute foods that are lower in calories and/or fat.

Serving size--8 ounces:	Calories kcal	Carbo grams	Prot grams	Fat grams	Fat % of kcal	Chol mg
Chicken back w/skin, batter fried	751	23.4	49.9	49.7	60	200
(chicken back meat, roasted)	542	0	64.0	29.9	50	204
Chicken back w/skin, flour fried	751	14.7	63.1	46.9	56	202
(chicken back meat, roasted)	542	0	64.0	29.9	50	204
Chicken back w/skin, roasted	680	0	58.7	47.6	63	200
(chicken back meat, roasted)	542	0	64.0	29.9	50	204
Chicken back w/skin, stewed	585	0	50.3	41.1	63	177
(chicken back meat, stewed)	474	0	57.4	25.4	48	193
Chicken breast, meat only, fried	424	1.1	75.8	10.7	23	206
(chicken breast, meat only, roasted)	374	0	70.3	8.2	20	193
Chicken breast, meat only, roasted	374	0	70.3	8.2	20	193
(fish, cod, unprepared)	186	0	40.3	1.6	8	97
Chicken breast, meat only, stewed	342	0	65.8	6.8	18	175
(fish, cod, unprepared)	186	0	40.3	1.6	8	97
Chicken breast w/skin batter fried	590	20.4	56.2	29.9	46	193
(chicken breast, meat only, roasted)	374	0	70.3	8.2	20	193
Chicken breast w/skin, flour fried	503	3.6	72.1	20.2	36	202
(chicken breast, meat only, roasted)	374	0	70.3	8.2	20	193
Chicken breast w/skin, roasted	447	0	67.6	17.7	36	191
(chicken breast, meat only, roasted)	374	0	70.3	8.2	20	193
Chicken breast w/skin, stewed	417	0	62.1	16.8	36	170
(chicken breast, meat only, stewed)	342	0	65.8	6.8	18	175
Chicken, canned with broth	374	0	49.4	17.9	43	141
(chicken breast, meat only, stewed)	342	0	65.8	6.8	18	175
Chicken chow mein, canned	86	16.1	5.9	0.2	2	7
(chicken gumbo soup)	52	7.7	2.5	1.4	24	3
Chicken chow mein, homemade	231	9.1	28.1	9.1	35	70
(chicken chow mein, canned)	86	16.1	5.9	0.2	2	7
Chicken cordon bleu	433	7.7	54.2	19.3	40	177
(chicken breast, meat only, roasted)	374	0	70.3	8.2	20	193
Chicken, dark meat, fried	542	5.9	65.8	26.3	44	218
(chicken breast, meat only, roasted)	374	0	70.3	8.2	20	193
Chicken, dark meat, roasted	465	0	62.1	22.0	43	211
(chicken breast, meat only, roasted)	374	0	70.3	8.2	20	193

( ) indicates possible substitute foods that are lower in calories and/or fat.

Serving size--8 ounces:	Calories kcal	Carbo grams	Prot grams	Fat grams	Fat % of kcal	Chol mg
Chicken, dark meat, stewed	435	0	59.0	20.4	42	200
(chicken breast, meat only, stewed)	342	0	65.8	6.8	18	175
Chicken, dark w/skin, batter fried	676	21.3	49.4	42.2	56	202
(chicken breast, meat only, roasted)	374	0	70.3	8.2	20	193
Chicken, dark w/skin, flour fried	646	9.3	61.7	38.3	53	209
(chicken breast, meat only, roasted)	374	0	70.3	8.2	20	193
Chicken, dark w/skin, roasted	574	0	59.0	35.8	56	206
(chicken breast, meat only, roasted)	374	0	70.3	8.2	20	193
Chicken, dark w/skin, stewed	528	0	53.3	33.3	57	186
(chicken breast, meat only, stewed)	342	0	65.8	6.8	18	175
Chicken dijon	438	2.9	58.5	20.4	42	161
(chicken breast, meat only, roasted)	374	0	70.3	8.2	20	193
Chicken drum, meat only, fried	442	0	64.9	18.4	37	213
(chicken drum, meat only, roasted)	390	0	64.2	12.9	30	211
Chicken drum, meat only, roasted	390	0	64.2	12.9	30	211
(chicken breast, meat only, roasted)	374	0	70.3	8.2	20	193
Chicken drum, meat only, stewed	383	0	62.4	12.9	30	200
(chicken breast, meat only, stewed)	342	0	65.8	6.8	18	175
Chicken drum w/skin, batter fried	608	18.8	49.7	35.8	53	195
(chicken drum, meat only, roasted)	390	0	64.2	12.9	30	211
Chicken drum w/skin, flour fried	556	3.6	61.2	31.1	50	204
(chicken drum, meat only, roasted)	390	0	64.2	12.9	30	211
Chicken drum w/skin, roasted	490	0	61.2	25.2	46	206
(chicken drum, meat only, roasted)	390	0	64.2	12.9	30	211
Chicken drum w/skin, stewed	463	0	57.4	24.0	47	188
(chicken drum, meat only, stewed)	383	0	62.4	12.9	30	200
Chicken enchiladas	678	82.8	29.7	24.5	33	82
(bean burrito)	426	63.7	14.7	12.9	27	16
Chicken fat	1427	0	8.4	154.0	97	132
(chicken breast, meat only, roasted)	374	0	70.3	8.2	20	193
Chicken frankfurter (hot dog)	583	15.4	29.3	44.2	68	229
(chicken breast, meat only, roasted)	374	0	70.3	8.2	20	193
Chicken fricassee	365	7.3	34.7	21.1	52	91
(chicken chow mein, canned)	86	16.1	5.9	0.2	2	7

( ) indicates possible substitute foods that are lower in calories and/or fat.

Serving size--8 ounces:	Calories kcal	Carbo grams	Prot grams	Fat grams	Fat % of kcal	Chol mg
Chicken giblets, fried	628	9.8	73.7	30.6	44	1012
(chicken giblets, simmered)	356	2.0	58.5	10.9	28	891
Chicken giblets, simmered	356	2.0	58.5	10.9	28	891
(chicken gizzard, simmered)	347	2.5	61.5	8.4	22	440
Chicken gizzard, simmered	347	2.5	61.5	8.4	22	440
(chicken breast, meat only, stewed)	342	0	65.8	6.8	18	175
Chicken heart, simmered	420	0.2	59.9	17.9	38	549
(chicken breast, meat only, roasted)	374	0	70.3	8.2	20	193
Chicken kiev	776	37.6	38.1	51.9	60	385
(chicken breast, meat only, roasted)	374	0	70.3	8.2	20	193
Chicken leg, meat only, fried	472	1.4	64.4	21.1	40	225
(chicken leg, meat only, roasted)	433	0	61.2	19.1	40	213
Chicken leg, meat only, roasted	433	0	61.2	19.1	40	213
(chicken breast, meat only, roasted)	374	0	70.3	8.2	20	193
Chicken leg, meat only, stewed	420	0	59.6	18.4	39	202
(chicken breast, meat only, stewed)	342	0	65.8	6.8	18	175
Chicken leg w/skin, batter fried	619	19.7	49.4	36.7	53	204
(chicken leg, meat only, roasted)	433	0	61.2	19.1	40	213
Chicken leg w/skin, flour fried	576	5.7	60.8	32.7	51	213
(chicken leg, meat only, roasted)	433	0	61.2	19.1	40	213
Chicken leg w/skin, roasted	526	0	59.0	30.6	52	209
(chicken leg, meat only, roasted)	433	0	61.2	19.1	40	213
Chicken leg w/skin, stewed	499	0	54.9	29.3	53	191
(chicken breast, meat only, stewed)	342	0	65.8	6.8	18	175
Chicken, light meat, fried	435	0.9	74.4	12.5	26	204
(chicken breast, meat only, roasted)	374	0	70.3	8.2	20	193
Chicken, light meat, roasted	392	0	70.1	10.2	23	193
(chicken breast, meat only, roasted)	374	0	70.3	8.2	20	193
Chicken, light meat, stewed	361	0	65.5	9.1	23	175
(chicken breast, meat only, stewed)	342	0	65.8	6.8	18	175
Chicken, light w/skin, batter fried	628	21.5	53.3	34.9	50	191
(chicken breast, meat only, roasted)	374	0	70.3	8.2	20	193
Chicken, light w/skin, flour fried	558	4.1	68.9	27.4	44	197
(chicken breast, meat only, roasted)	374	0	70.3	8.2	20	193

( ) indicates possible substitute foods that are lower in calories and/or fat.

Serving size--8 ounces:	Calories kcal	Carbo grams	Prot grams	Fat grams	Fat % of kcal	Chol mg
Chicken, light w/skin, roasted	503	0	65.8	24.5	44	191
(chicken breast, meat only, roasted)	374	0	70.3	8.2	20	193
Chicken liver pate	456	14.7	30.4	29.7	59	887
(chicken spread, canned)	435	12.2	34.9	26.5	55	118
Chicken liver, simmered	356	2.0	55.3	12.2	31	1431
(chicken gizzard, simmered)	347	2.5	61.5	8.4	22	440
Chicken meat/skin, batter fried	655	21.3	51.0	39.2	54	197
(chicken breast, meat only, roasted)	374	0	70.3	8.2	20	193
Chicken meat/skin, flour fried	610	7.0	64.9	33.8	50	204
(chicken breast, meat only, roasted)	374	0	70.3	8.2	20	193
Chicken meat/skin, roasted	542	0	61.9	30.8	51	200
(chicken breast, meat only, roasted)	374	0	70.3	8.2	20	193
Chicken meat/skin, stewed	497	0	56.0	28.6	52	177
(chicken breast, meat only, stewed)	342	0	65.8	6.8	18	175
Chicken, meat only, fried	497	3.9	69.4	20.6	37	213
(chicken breast, meat only, roasted)	374	0	70.3	8.2	20	193
Chicken, meat only, roasted	431	0	65.5	16.8	35	202
(chicken breast, meat only, roasted)	374	0	70.3	8.2	20	193
Chicken, meat only, stewed	401	0	61.9	15.2	34	188
(chicken breast, meat only, stewed)	342	0	65.8	6.8	18	175
Chicken neck, meat only, fried	519	4.1	61.0	27.0	47	238
(chicken neck, meat only, stewed)	406	0	55.8	18.6	41	179
Chicken neck, meat only, stewed	406	0	55.8	18.6	41	179
(chicken breast, meat only, stewed)	342	0	65.8	6.8	18	175
Chicken neck w/skin, batter fried	748	19.7	44.9	53.3	64	206
(chicken neck, meat only, stewed)	406	0	55.8	18.6	41	179
Chicken neck w/skin, flour fried	753	9.5	54.4	53.5	64	213
(chicken neck, meat only, stewed)	406	0	55.8	18.6	41	179
Chicken neck w/skin, stewed	560	0	44.5	41.1	66	159
(chicken neck, meat only, stewed)	406	0	55.8	18.6	41	179
Chicken parmesan	465	16.8	40.8	25.6	50	131
(chicken breast, meat only, roasted)	374	0	70.3	8.2	20	193
Chicken pot pie, frozen, cooked	497	50.3	15.2	26.1	47	29
(chicken chow mein, canned)	86	16.1	5.9	0.2	2	7

( ) indicates possible substitute foods that are lower in calories and/or fat.

Pltry

Serving size--8 ounces:	Calories kcal	Carbo grams	Prot grams	Fat grams	Fat % of kcal	Chol mg
Chicken potpie, homemade	533	41.5	22.9	30.6	52	70
(chicken chow mein, canned)	86	16.1	5.9	0.2	2	7
Chicken roll, light	361	5.4	44.2	16.8	42	113
(turkey loaf breast)	249	0	51.0	3.6	13	93
Chicken salad sandwich	694	33.3	43.1	42.2	55	139
(grilled chicken sandwich)	474	40.1	53.1	9.8	19	133
Chicken skin, batter fried	894	52.4	23.4	65.3	66	168
(chicken breast, meat only, roasted)	374	0	70.3	8.2	20	193
Chicken skin, flour fried	1139	21.1	43.3	96.6	76	166
(chicken breast, meat only, roasted)	374	0	70.3	8.2	20	193
Chicken skin, roasted	1030	0	46.3	92.3	81	188
(chicken breast, meat only, roasted)	374	0	70.3	8.2	20	193
Chicken skin, stewed	823	0	34.5	74.8	82	143
(chicken breast, meat only, stewed)	342	0	65.8	6.8	18	175
Chicken spread, canned	435	12.2	34.9	26.5	55	118
(chicken breast, meat only, roasted)	374	0	70.3	8.2	20	193
Chicken thigh, meat only, fried	494	2.7	64.0	23.4	43	231
(chicken breast, meat only, roasted)	374	0	70.3	8.2	20	193
Chicken thigh, meat only, roasted	474	0	58.7	24.7	47	215
(chicken breast, meat only, roasted)	374	0	70.3	8.2	20	193
Chicken thigh, meat only, stewed	442	0	56.7	22.2	45	204
(chicken breast, meat only, stewed)	342	0	65.8	6.8	18	175
Chicken thigh w/skin, batter fried	628	20.6	49.0	37.4	54	211
(chicken thigh, meat only, roasted)	474	0	58.7	24.7	47	215
Chicken thigh w/skin, flour fried	594	7.3	60.8	34.0	52	220
(chicken thigh, meat only, roasted)	474	0	58.7	24.7	47	215
Chicken thigh w/skin, roasted	560	0	56.9	35.2	57	211
(chicken thigh, meat only, roasted)	474	0	58.7	24.7	47	215
Chicken thigh w/skin, stewed	526	0	52.8	33.3	57	191
(chicken thigh, meat only, stewed)	442	0	56.7	22.2	45	204
Chicken, whole, batter fried	660	20.4	51.7	39.7	54	234
(chicken breast, meat only, roasted)	374	0	70.3	8.2	20	193
Chicken, whole, flour fried	617	7.5	64.9	34.7	51	254
(chicken breast, meat only, roasted)	374	0	70.3	8.2	20	193

( ) indicates possible substitute foods that are lower in calories and/or fat.

Serving size--8 ounces:	Calories kcal	Carbo grams	Prot grams	Fat grams	Fat % of kcal	Chol mg
Chicken, whole, roasted	530	0	60.7	30.1	51	242
(chicken breast, meat only, roasted)	374	0	70.3	8.2	20	193
Chicken, whole, stewed	625	0	55.5	28.1	53	220
(chicken breast, meat only, stewed)	342	0	65.8	6.8	18	175
Chicken wing, meat only, fried	479	0	68.3	20.6	39	191
(chicken breast, meat only, roasted)	374	0	70.3	8.2	20	193
Chicken wing, meat only, roasted	460	0	69.2	18.4	36	193
(chicken breast, meat only, roasted)	374	0	70.3	8.2	20	193
Chicken wing, meat only, stewed	411	0	61.7	16.3	36	168
(chicken breast, meat only, stewed)	342	0	65.8	6.8	18	175
Chicken wing w/skin, batter fried	735	24.7	45.1	49.4	60	179
(chicken wing, meat only, roasted)	460	0	69.2	18.4	36	193
Chicken wing w/skin, flour fried	728	5.4	59.2	50.3	62	184
(chicken wing, meat only, roasted)	460	0	69.2	18.4	36	193
Chicken wing w/skin, roasted	658	0	61.0	44.2	60	191
(chicken wing, meat only, roasted)	460	0	69.2	18.4	36	193
Chicken wing w/skin, stewed	565	0	51.7	38.1	61	159
(chicken wing, meat only, stewed)	411	0	61.7	16.3	36	168
Duck fat	2041	0	0	226.3	100	227
(duck, meat only, roasted)	456	0	53.3	25.4	50	202
Duck liver	308	7.9	42.4	10.4	30	1168
(goose liver)	302	14.3	37.2	9.8	29	1168
Duck, meat only, roasted	456	0	53.3	25.4	50	202
(wild duck, breast meat)	279	0	44.9	9.8	32	175
Duck meat with skin, roasted	764	0	43.1	64.2	76	191
(wild duck, breast meat)	279	0	44.9	9.8	32	175
Goose fat	2041	0	0	226.3	100	227
(goose meat with skin, roasted)	692	0	57.2	49.7	65	206
Goose liver	302	14.3	37.2	9.8	29	1168
(guinea, meat only)	249	0	46.7	5.7	21	143
Goose liver pate	1048	10.7	25.9	99.3	85	340
(chicken spread, canned)	435	12.2	34.9	26.5	55	118
Goose, meat only, roasted	540	0	65.8	28.8	48	218
(chicken breast, meat only, roasted)	374	0	70.3	8.2	20	193

( ) indicates possible substitute foods that are lower in calories and/or fat.

Serving size--8 ounces:	Calories kcal	Carbo grams	Prot grams	Fat grams	Fat % of kcal	Chol mg
Goose meat with skin, roasted	692	0	57.2	49.7	65	206
(goose, meat only, roasted)	540	0	65.8	28.8	48	218
Guinea, meat only	249	0	46.7	5.7	21	143
(fish, cod, unprepared)	186	0	40.3	1.6	8	97
Guinea meat with skin	358	0	53.1	14.5	36	168
(guinea, meat only)	249	0	46.7	5.7	21	143
Pheasant, breast meat	302	0	55.3	7.5	22	132
(guinea, meat only)	249	0	46.7	5.7	21	143
Pheasant, leg meat	304	0	50.3	9.8	29	181
(guinea, meat only)	249	0	46.7	5.7	21	143
Pheasant, meat only	302	0	53.5	8.2	24	150
(guinea, meat only)	249	0	46.7	5.7	21	143
Pheasant meat with skin	411	0	51.5	21.1	46	161
(pheasant, breast meat)	302	0	55.3	7.5	22	132
Poultry salad spread	454	16.8	26.3	30.6	61	68
(tuna salad)	424	21.3	36.3	21.1	45	29
Quail, breast meat	279	0	51.3	6.8	22	132
(guinea, meat only)	249	0	46.7	5.7	21	143
Quail, meat only	304	0	49.4	10.2	30	159
(quail, breast meat)	279	0	51.3	6.8	22	132
Quail meat with skin	435	0	44.5	27.2	56	172
(quail, breast meat)	279	0	51.3	6.8	22	132
Squab, breast meat	304	0	49.4	10.2	30	204
(guinea, meat only)	249	0	46.7	5.7	21	143
Squab, meat only	322	0	39.7	17.0	48	204
(squab, breast meat)	304	0	49.4	10.2	30	204
Squab meat with skin	667	0	42.0	54.0	73	215
(squab, breast meat)	304	0	49.4	10.2	30	204
Turkey back with skin, roasted	551	0	60.3	32.7	53	206
(turkey, light, meat only, roasted)	356	0	67.8	7.3	18	156
Turkey bacon	934	26.8	80.1	53.3	51	267
(ham, canned, extra-lean)	308	1.1	48.0	11.1	34	68
Turkey bologna	451	2.3	31.1	34.5	69	225
(turkey loaf breast)	249	0	51.0	3.6	13	93

( ) indicates possible substitute foods that are lower in calories and/or fat.

Serving size--8 ounces:	Calories kcal	Carbo grams	Prot grams	Fat grams	Fat % of kcal	Chol mg
Turkey breast with skin, roasted	429	0	65.1	16.8	35	168
(turkey, light, meat only, roasted)	356	0	67.8	7.3	18	156
Turkey fat	2041	0	0	226.3	100	231
(turkey, light, meat only, roasted)	356	0	67.8	7.3	18	156
Turkey frankfurter (hot dog)	513	3.4	32.4	40.1	70	243
(turkey, light, meat only, roasted)	356	0	67.8	7.3	18	156
Turkey giblets, simmered	379	4.8	60.3	11.6	28	948
(turkey, light, meat only, roasted)	356	0	67.8	7.3	18	156
Turkey gizzard, simmered	370	1.4	66.7	8.8	21	526
(turkey, light, meat only, roasted)	356	0	67.8	7.3	18	156
Turkey heart, simmered	401	4.5	60.8	13.8	31	513
(turkey, light, meat only, roasted)	356	0	67.8	7.3	18	156
Turkey leg with skin, roasted	472	0	63.3	22.2	42	193
(turkey, light, meat only, roasted)	356	0	67.8	7.3	18	156
Turkey, light, meat only, roasted	356	0	67.8	7.3	18	156
(turkey loaf breast)	249	0	51.0	3.6	13	93
Turkey, light with skin, roasted	447	0	64.9	18.8	38	172
(turkey, light, meat only, roasted)	356	0	67.8	7.3	18	156
Turkey liver, simmered	383	7.7	54.4	13.4	31	1420
(turkey, light, meat only, roasted)	356	0	67.8	7.3	18	156
Turkey loaf breast	249	0	51.0	3.6	13	93
(fish, cod, unprepared)	186	0	40.3	1.6	8	97
Turkey, meat only, roasted	386	0	66.5	11.3	26	172
(turkey, light, meat only, roasted)	356	0	67.8	7.3	18	156
Turkey meat with skin, roasted	472	0	63.7	22.0	42	186
(turkey, light, meat only, roasted)	356	0	67.8	7.3	18	156
Turkey neck meat, simmered	408	0	60.8	16.6	37	277
(turkey, light, meat only, roasted)	356	0	67.8	7.3	18	156
Turkey pastrami	320	3.9	41.7	14.1	40	122
(turkey loaf breast)	249	0	51.0	3.6	13	93
Turkey patty, breaded, fried	642	35.6	31.8	40.8	57	141
(turkey, light, meat only, roasted)	356	0	67.8	7.3	18	156
Turkey roast, light/dark	352	7.0	48.3	13.2	34	120
(turkey loaf breast)	249	0	51.0	3.6	13	93

( ) indicates possible substitute foods that are lower in calories and/or fat.

Serving size--8 ounces:	Calories kcal	Carbo grams	Prot grams	Fat grams	Fat % of kcal	Chol mg
Turkey roll, light	333	1.1	42.4	16.3	44	98
(turkey loaf breast)	249	0	51.0	3.6	13	93
Turkey roll, light/dark	338	4.8	41.1	15.9	42	125
(turkey loaf breast)	249	0	51.0	3.6	13	93
Turkey salami	445	1.1	37.2	31.3	63	186
(turkey loaf breast)	249	0	51.0	3.6	13	93
Turkey sandwich	401	47.6	36.3	4.5	11	54
(chicken and rice casserole)	258	34.4	18.1	4.8	17	47
Turkey sandwich w/mayonnaise	569	36.1	47.9	24.7	39	121
(turkey sandwich)	401	47.6	36.3	4.5	11	54
Turkey skin roasted	1002	0	44.7	90.0	81	256
(turkey, light, meat only, roasted)	356	0	67.8	7.3	18	156
Turkey stick, breaded, fried	633	38.6	32.2	38.3	54	145
(turkey, light, meat only, roasted)	356	0	67.8	7.3	18	156
Turkey wing with skin, roasted	519	0	62.1	28.1	49	184
(turkey, light, meat only, roasted)	356	0	67.8	7.3	18	156
Whole capon, roasted	513	0	64.2	26.5	46	234
(chicken breast, meat only, roasted)	374	0	70.3	8.2	20	193
Whole turkey, roasted	465	0.2	63.5	21.3	41	215
(turkey, light, meat only, roasted)	356	0	67.8	7.3	18	156

( ) indicates possible substitute foods that are lower in calories and/or fat.

SALAD DRESSINGS, OILS AND FATS

The serving size used for salad dressings, oils and fats is 0.5 ounce. This serving size roughly equates to one tablespoon.

Weights and Measures

1. One stick of butter or margarine (4 sticks per pound) weighs four ounces.
2. One tablespoon of most salad dressings, oils and fats weighs approximately one-half ounce.

Serving size--0.5 ounce:	Calories kcal	Carbo grams	Prot grams	Fat grams	Fat % of kcal	Chol mg
Blue cheese salad dressing	71	1.0	0.7	7.4	94	2
(fat-free blue cheese salad dressing)	20	4.0	0	0	0	0
Coconut oil	125	0	0	14.2	100	0
(promise ultra fat-free margarine)	5	0	0	0	0	0
Corn oil	125	0	0	14.2	100	0
(promise ultra fat-free margarine)	5	0	0	0	0	0
Cottonseed oil	125	0	0	14.2	100	0
(promise ultra fat-free margarine)	5	0	0	0	0	0
Fat-free blue cheese salad dressing	20	4.0	0	0	0	0
(fat-free italian low-cal dressing)	4	0.6	0	0	0	0
Fat-free catalina low-cal dressing	32	6.0	0	0	0	0
(fat-free italian low-cal dressing)	4	0.6	0	0	0	0
Fat-free french low-cal dressing	40	8.0	0	0	0	0
(fat-free italian low-cal dressing)	4	0.6	0	0	0	0
Fat-free italian low-cal dressing	4	0.6	0	0	0	0
(vinegar)	2	0.8	0	0	0	0
Fat-free mayonnaise	10	2.0	0	0	0	0
(mexican salsa)	3	0.7	0.1	0	0	0
Fat-free miracle whip	14	2.8	0	0	0	0
(fat-free italian low-cal dressing)	4	0.6	0	0	0	0
Fat-free ranch low-cal dressing	32	6.0	0	0	0	0
(fat-free italian low-cal dressing)	4	0.6	0	0	0	0

( ) indicates possible substitute foods that are lower in calories and/or fat.

Serving size--0.5 ounce:	Calories kcal	Carbo grams	Prot grams	Fat grams	Fat % of kcal	Chol mg
Fat-free thousand island dressing	40	10	0	0	0	0
(fat-free italian low-cal dressing)	4	0.6	0	0	0	0
Fat, lard	128	0	0	14.2	100	13
(promise ultra fat-free margarine)	5	0	0	0	0	0
French salad dressing	61	2.5	0.1	5.8	86	8
(fat-free french low-cal dressing)	40	8.0	0	0	0	0
Grape-seed oil	125	0	0	14.2	100	0
(promise ultra fat-free margarine)	5	0	0	0	0	0
Hard margarine	102	0.1	0.1	11.4	99	0
(promise ultra fat-free margarine)	5	0	0	0	0	0
Hazelnut oil	125	0	0	14.2	100	0
(promise ultra fat-free margarine)	5	0	0	0	0	0
Imitation margarine	49	0.1	0.1	5.5	98	0
(promise ultra fat-free margarine)	5	0	0	0	0	0
Imitation mayonnaise, no chol	68	2.2	0	6.8	90	0
(fat-free mayonnaise)	10	2.0	0	0	0	0
Italian salad dressing	66	1.4	0.1	6.8	93	0
(fat-free italian low-cal dressing)	4	0.6	0	0	0	0
Linseed oil	125	0	0	14.2	100	0
(promise ultra fat-free margarine)	5	0	0	0	0	0
Liquid margarine	102	0	0.3	11.4	99	0
(promise ultra fat-free margarine)	5	0	0	0	0	0
Low-cal french salad dressing	19	3.1	0	0.8	38	1
(fat-free french low-cal dressing)	14	3.0	0	0	0	0
Low-cal italian salad dressing	15	0.7	0	1.4	84	1
(fat-free low-cal italian dressing)	4	0.6	0	0	0	0
Low-cal russian salad dressing	20	3.9	0.1	0.6	27	1
(fat-free low-cal italian dressing)	4	0.6	0	0	0	0
Low-cal thousand island dressing	23	2.3	0.1	1.5	59	2
(low-cal russian salad dressing)	20	3.9	0.1	0.6	27	1
Mayonnaise	102	0.4	0.2	11.3	98	8
(fat-free mayonnaise)	10	2.0	0	0	0	0
Mayonnaise-type salad dressing	55	3.4	0.1	4.7	77	4
(fat-free mayonnaise)	10	2.0	0	0	0	0

( ) indicates possible substitute foods that are lower in calories and/or fat.

Serving size--0.5 ounce:	Calories kcal	Carbo grams	Prot grams	Fat grams	Fat % of kcal	Chol mg
Miracle whip	70	2.0	0	7.0	90	6
(fat-free miracle whip)	14	2.8	0	0	0	0
Miracle whip light	42	2.0	0	4.0	86	6
(fat-free miracle whip)	14	2.8	0	0	0	0
Olive oil	125	0	0	14.2	100	0
(promise ultra fat-free margarine)	5	0	0	0	0	0
Palm oil	125	0	0	14.2	100	0
(promise ultra fat-free margarine)	5	0	0	0	0	0
Peanut oil	125	0	0	14.2	100	0
(promise ultra fat-free margarine)	5	0	0	0	0	0
Poppyseed oil	125	0	0	14.2	100	0
(promise ultra fat-free margarine)	5	0	0	0	0	0
Promise ultra fat-free margarine	5	0	0	0	0	0
(canned au jus gravy)	2	0.4	0.2	0	0	0
Russian salad dressing, regular	70	1.5	0.2	7.2	93	3
(low-cal russian salad dressing)	20	3.9	0.1	0.6	27	1
Safflower oil	125	0	0	14.2	100	0
(promise ultra fat-free margarine)	5	0	0	0	0	0
Sandwich spread	55	3.2	0.1	4.8	79	11
(fat-free mayonnaise)	10	2.0	0	0	0	0
Sesame oil	125	0	0	14.2	100	0
(promise ultra fat-free margarine)	5	0	0	0	0	0
Sesame seed salad dressing	63	1.2	0.4	6.4	91	0
(fat-free low-cal italian dressing)	4	0.6	0	0	0	0
Shortening	125	0	0	14.2	100	0
(promise ultra fat-free margarine)	5	0	0	0	0	0
Soft margarine	101	0.1	0.1	11.4	99	0
(promise ultra fat-free margarine)	5	0	0	0	0	0
Soybean oil	125	0	0	14.2	100	0
(promise ultra fat-free margarine)	5	0	0	0	0	0
Sunflower oil	125	0	0	14.2	100	0
(promise ultra fat-free margarine)	5	0	0	0	0	0
Thousand island salad dressing	53	2.2	0.1	5.1	87	4
(fat-free thousand island dressing)	40	10	0	0	0	0

( ) indicates possible substitute foods that are lower in calories and/or fat.

Serving size--0.5 ounce:	Calories kcal	Carbo grams	Prot grams	Fat grams	Fat % of kcal	Chol mg
Tomato-seed oil	125	0	0	14.2	100	0
(promise ultra fat-free margarine)	5	0	0	0	0	0
Vegetable oil	125	0	0	14.2	100	0
(promise ultra fat-free margarine)	5	0	0	0	0	0
Vinegar	2	0.8	0	0	0	0
(no alternate identified)						
Vinegar and oil salad dressing	64	0.4	0	7.1	98	0
(fat-free low-cal italian dressing)	4	0.6	0	0	0	0
Walnut oil	125	0	0	14.2	100	0
(promise ultra fat-free margarine)	5	0	0	0	0	0

( ) indicates possible substitute foods that are lower in calories and/or fat.

SANDWICHES

The serving size used for Sandwiches is 4 ounces. Because sandwiches vary in their weight and content depending upon the ratio of ingredients (e.g., meat versus lettuce versus tomato, etc.), you may wish to analyze the individual components of your sandwich to obtain a more accurate analysis of its nutritional content. Also, please note that the caloric and fat content of your sandwich may vary significantly depending upon which condiments you use. (See Sauces, Gravy and Condiments.)

Weights and Measures

1. Two slices of bread weigh approximately two ounces.
2. One slice of cheese (3 1/2" x 3 3/8" x 1/8") weighs approximately one ounce.
3. One slice of lunch meat weighs approximately one ounce (e.g., one-pound package of bologna cut into 16 slices).
4. One fast food hamburger/cheeseburger (e.g., McDonald's, Burger King) weighs approximately four ounces.
5. One McDonald's Quarter Pounder weighs approximately six ounces.
6. One fast food regular roast beef (e.g., Arby's, Rax) weighs approximately five ounces.
7. One tablespoon of condiments weighs approximately one-half ounce.

Serving size--4 ounces:	Calories kcal	Carbo grams	Prot grams	Fat grams	Fat % of kcal	Chol mg
Bacon cheeseburger	435	15.2	24.7	30.1	62	80
(grilled chicken sandwich)	237	20.1	26.5	4.9	19	67
Bacon cheeseburger w/mayonnaise	447	13.7	22.9	32.9	66	78
(grilled chicken sandwich)	237	20.1	26.5	4.9	19	67
Bacon, lettuce and tomato sandwich	260	24.4	11.2	12.6	44	21
(turkey breast sandwich)	201	23.8	18.1	2.3	10	27
Bacon, lettuce and tomato w/mayo	310	22.5	10.3	19.7	57	25
(turkey breast sandwich)	201	23.8	18.1	2.3	10	27
Cheese sandwich	414	20.4	22.6	26.8	58	82
(turkey breast sandwich)	201	23.8	18.1	2.3	10	27

( ) indicates possible substitute foods that are lower in calories and/or fat.

Serving size--4 ounces:	Calories kcal	Carbo grams	Prot grams	Fat grams	Fat % of kcal	Chol mg
Cheese sandwich w/mayonnaise	449	18.9	20.8	32.2	65	81
(turkey breast sandwich)	201	23.8	18.1	2.3	10	27
Cheeseburger on bun, plain	352	15.1	22.9	21.7	55	82
(grilled chicken sandwich)	237	20.1	26.5	4.9	19	67
Cheeseburger w/cond.,veg	264	20.8	13.2	14.5	49	39
(grilled chicken sandwich)	237	20.1	26.5	4.9	19	67
Cheeseburger w/mayonnaise	367	13.5	21.2	25.1	62	80
(grilled chicken sandwich)	237	20.1	26.5	4.9	19	67
Chicken fillet sandwich, plain	321	24.2	15.1	18.4	52	37
(grilled chicken sandwich)	237	20.1	26.5	4.9	19	67
Chicken salad sandwich	347	16.7	21.5	21.1	55	70
(grilled chicken sandwich)	237	20.1	26.5	4.9	19	67
Cold cut submarine sandwich	227	25.4	10.9	9.3	37	18
(turkey breast sandwich)	201	23.8	18.1	2.3	10	27
Corned beef sandwich	390	19.4	21.0	24.6	57	74
(turkey breast sandwich)	201	23.8	18.1	2.3	10	27
Corned beef sandwich w/mayonnaise	426	18.0	19.4	30.3	64	73
(turkey breast sandwich)	201	23.8	18.1	2.3	10	27
Fish sandwich, plain	279	24.6	18.0	11.5	37	46
(grilled chicken sandwich)	237	20.1	26.5	4.9	19	67
Fish sandwich, tartar sauce&cheese	324	29.5	12.8	17.7	49	42
(grilled chicken sandwich)	237	20.1	26.5	4.9	19	67
Fish sandwich with tartar sauce	310	29.5	12.1	16.3	47	40
(grilled chicken sandwich)	237	20.1	26.5	4.9	19	67
Grilled cheese sandwich	384	29.3	17.4	22.0	52	55
(grilled chicken sandwich)	237	20.1	26.5	4.9	19	67
Grilled chicken sandwich	237	20.1	26.5	4.9	19	67
(chicken and rice casserole)	129	17.2	9.1	2.4	17	23
Ham and cheese w/mayonnaise	372	13.9	23.2	24.3	59	79
(ham sandwich)	330	19.4	22.6	17.2	47	73
Ham and swiss cheese	356	15.5	25.2	20.9	53	81
(turkey breast sandwich)	201	23.8	18.1	2.3	10	27
Ham sandwich	330	19.4	22.6	17.2	47	73
(turkey breast sandwich)	201	23.8	18.1	2.3	10	27

( ) indicates possible substitute foods that are lower in calories and/or fat.

Serving size--4 ounces:	Calories kcal	Carbo grams	Prot grams	Fat grams	Fat % of kcal	Chol mg
Ham sandwich w/mayonnaise	372	18.0	20.9	23.4	57	72
(turkey breast sandwich)	201	23.8	18.1	2.3	10	27
Hamburger on bun, plain	324	19.4	22.0	16.9	47	74
(grilled chicken sandwich)	237	20.1	26.5	4.9	19	67
Hamburger w/cheese and mayonnaise	367	13.5	21.2	25.1	62	80
(grilled chicken sandwich)	237	20.1	26.5	4.9	19	67
Hamburger w/cheese, bacon & mayo	447	13.7	22.9	32.9	66	78
(grilled chicken sandwich)	237	20.1	26.5	4.9	19	67
Hamburger w/mayonnaise	366	18.0	20.3	23.1	57	73
(grilled chicken sandwich)	237	20.1	26.5	4.9	19	67
Hamburger with cheese	352	15.1	22.9	21.7	55	82
(grilled chicken sandwich)	237	20.1	26.5	4.9	19	67
Hamburger with cheese and bacon	435	15.2	24.7	30.1	62	80
(grilled chicken sandwich)	237	20.1	26.5	4.9	19	67
Hot dog on bun, plain	352	21.3	12.0	23.9	61	38
(grilled chicken sandwich)	237	20.1	26.5	4.9	19	67
Hot dog on bun with chili	295	31.1	13.4	13.4	41	51
(grilled chicken sandwich)	237	20.1	26.5	4.9	19	67
Hot dog w/sauerkraut & ketchup	256	17.0	8.7	16.9	59	27
(turkey breast sandwich)	201	23.8	18.1	2.3	10	27
Lobster salad sandwich	188	21.2	11.1	6.1	29	37
(lobster, spiny)	127	2.7	23.4	1.7	13	80
Pastrami sandwich	212	20.8	17.6	6.0	25	43
(turkey breast sandwich)	201	23.8	18.1	2.3	10	27
Pastrami sandwich w/mayonnaise	264	19.3	16.2	13.2	45	45
(turkey breast sandwich)	201	23.8	18.1	2.3	10	27
Peanut butter and jelly sandwich	375	53.4	12.2	13.6	33	2
(turkey breast sandwich)	201	23.8	18.1	2.3	10	27
Reuben sandwich	295	15.4	15.1	19.2	59	53
(turkey breast sandwich)	201	23.8	18.1	2.3	10	27
Roast beef sandwich	277	19.4	22.6	11.2	36	71
(turkey breast sandwich)	201	23.8	18.1	2.3	10	27
Roast beef sandwich w/mayonnaise	322	18.0	20.9	17.9	50	71
(turkey breast sandwich)	201	23.8	18.1	2.3	10	27

( ) indicates possible substitute foods that are lower in calories and/or fat.

Serving size--4 ounces:	Calories kcal	Carbo grams	Prot grams	Fat grams	Fat % of kcal	Chol mg
Roast beef submarine	215	23.2	15.1	6.8	28	39
(turkey breast sandwich)	201	23.8	18.1	2.3	10	27
Tuna salad sandwich	235	22.1	14.6	9.3	36	51
(tuna fish, canned in water)	144	0	31.8	0.9	6	71
Tuna salad submarine sandwich	259	24.5	13.2	12.4	43	22
(tuna salad sandwich)	235	22.1	14.6	9.3	36	51
Turkey club sandwich	401	15.2	26.2	25.6	57	75
(turkey breast sandwich)	201	23.8	18.1	2.3	10	27
Turkey club sandwich w/mayonnaise	415	13.7	24.3	28.8	62	73
(turkey breast sandwich)	201	23.8	18.1	2.3	10	27
Turkey breast sandwich	201	23.8	18.1	2.3	10	27
(chicken and rice casserole)	129	17.2	9.1	2.4	17	23
Turkey sandwich w/mayonnaise	285	18.0	23.9	12.4	39	60
(turkey breast sandwich)	201	23.8	18.1	2.3	10	27

( ) indicates possible substitute foods that are lower in calories and/or fat.

SAUCES, GRAVY AND CONDIMENTS

The serving size used for this category is 0.5 ounce. For most items in this food category, 0.5 ounce equates to approximately 1 tablespoon.

Serving size--0.5 ounce:	Calories kcal	Carbo grams	Prot grams	Fat grams	Fat % of kcal	Chol mg
Bearnaise sauce	39	1.0	0.5	3.8	85	10
(canned mushroom gravy)	7	0.8	0.2	0.4	51	0
Brown mustard	13	0.8	0.8	0.9	62	0
(ready-to-serve teriyaki sauce)	12	2.3	0.8	0	0	0
Canned au jus gravy	2	0.4	0.2	0	0	0
(dehydrated beef bouillon prepared)	<1	0	0	0	26	0
Canned beef gravy	8	0.7	0.5	0.3	34	0
(canned au jus gravy)	2	0.4	0.2	0	0	0
Canned chicken gravy	11	0.8	0.3	0.8	65	0
(canned turkey gravy)	7	0.7	0.4	0.3	39	0
Canned mushroom gravy	7	0.8	0.2	0.4	51	0
(canned au jus gravy)	2	0.4	0.2	0	0	0
Canned turkey gravy	7	0.7	0.4	0.3	39	0
(canned au jus gravy)	2	0.4	0.2	0	0	0
Chili sauce, hot, green	3	0.7	0.1	0	0	0
(vinegar)	2	0.8	0	0	0	0
Chili sauce, hot, red	3	0.6	0.1	0.1	22	0
(chili sauce, hot, green)	3	0.7	0.1	0	4	0
Chunky tomato sauce	5	1.0	0.2	0.1	18	0
(tomato sauce, canned)	4	1.0	0.2	0	0	0
Cocktail sauce	14	3.3	0.3	0.1	6	0
(Mexican salsa)	3	0.7	0.1	0	0	0
Diet sandwich spread	16	1.1	0.1	1.3	73	7
(tomato ketchup)	15	3.6	0.3	0.1	6	0
Dietary tartar sauce	32	0.9	0.1	3.2	90	7
(tomato ketchup)	15	3.6	0.3	0.1	6	0
Fat-free mayonnaise	10	2.0	0	0	0	0
(mexican salsa)	3	0.7	0.1	0	0	0

( ) indicates possible substitute foods that are lower in calories and/or fat.

Serving size--0.5 ounce:	Calories kcal	Carbo grams	Prot grams	Fat grams	Fat % of kcal	Chol mg
Fat-free miracle whip	14	2.8	0	0	0	0
(fat-free italian low-cal dressing)	4	0.6	0	0	0	0
Guacamole dip	24	0.9	0.3	2.3	86	0
(mexican salsa)	3	0.7	0.1	0	0	0
Horseradish, prepared	5	1.4	0.2	0	0	0
(chili sauce, hot, green)	3	0.7	0.1	0	4	0
Marinara sauce, canned	10	1.4	0.2	0.5	45	0
(ready-to-serve soy sauce)	9	1.2	1.2	0	0	0
Mayonnaise	102	0.4	0.2	11.3	98	8
(fat-free mayonnaise)	10	2.0	0	0	0	0
Mexican salsa	3	0.7	0.1	0	0	0
(canned au jus gravy)	2	0.4	0.2	0	0	0
Miracle whip	70	2.0	0	7.0	90	6
(fat-free miracle whip)	14	2.8	0	0	0	0
Miracle whip light	42	2.0	0	4.0	86	6
(fat-free miracle whip)	14	2.8	0	0	0	0
Pickle relish, sour	3	0.4	0.1	0.1	30	0
(canned au jus gravy)	2	0.4	0.2	0	0	0
Pickle relish, sweet	20	4.8	0.1	0.1	4	0
(pickle relish, sour)	3	0.4	0.1	0.1	30	0
Ready-to-serve barbecue sauce	11	1.8	0.3	0.3	25	0
(ready-to-serve soy sauce)	9	1.2	1.2	0	0	0
Ready-to-serve soy sauce	9	1.2	1.2	0	0	0
(canned au jus gravy)	2	0.4	0.2	0	0	0
Ready-to-serve teriyaki sauce	12	2.3	0.8	0	0	0
(tomato sauce, canned)	4	1.0	0.2	0	0	0
Red clam sauce	5	0.9	0.4	0	0	1
(tomato sauce, canned)	4	1.0	0.2	0	0	0
Sour cream & onion dip (chip dip)	31	1.2	0.6	2.8	81	6
(mexican salsa)	3	0.7	0.1	0	0	0
Spaghetti sauce canned	15	2.3	0.3	0.6	36	0
(tomato sauce, canned)	4	1.0	0.2	0	0	0
Tartar sauce	75	0.6	0.2	8.2	97	7
(dietary tartar sauce)	32	0.9	0.1	3.2	90	7

( ) indicates possible substitute foods that are lower in calories and/or fat.

Serving size--0.5 ounce:	Calories kcal	Carbo grams	Prot grams	Fat grams	Fat % of kcal	Chol mg
Tomato chile sauce	15	3.5	0.4	0	0	0
(tomato sauce, canned)	4	1.0	0.2	0	0	0
Tomato ketchup	15	3.6	0.3	0.1	6	0
(ready-to-serve teriyaki sauce)	12	2.3	0.8	0	0	0
Tomato sauce, canned	4	1.0	0.2	0	0	0
(mexican salsa)	3	0.7	0.1	0	0	0
Tomato sauce with mushroom	5	1.2	0.2	0	0	0
(tomato sauce, canned)	4	1.0	0.2	0	0	0
Tomato sauce with onions	6	1.4	0.2	0	0	0
(tomato sauce, canned)	4	1.0	0.2	0	0	0
White clam sauce	23	1.3	0.7	1.7	67	6
(red clam sauce)	5	0.9	0.4	0	0	1
White sauce, medium	23	1.2	0.6	1.8	70	6
(white sauce, thin)	17	1.0	0.6	1.2	64	4
White sauce, thick	28	1.6	0.6	2.2	71	7
(white sauce, thin)	17	1.0	0.6	1.2	64	4
White sauce, thin	17	1.0	0.6	1.2	64	4
(tomato sauce, canned)	4	1.0	0.2	0	0	0
Yellow mustard	11	0.9	0.7	0.6	49	0
(horseradish, prepared)	5	1.4	0.2	0	0	0

Sauce

( ) indicates possible substitute foods that are lower in calories and/or fat.

SEAFOOD

Because seafood, when it is served, is commonly a main dish, the serving size used for this category is 8 ounces.

Weights and Measures

1. One swordfish steak (4.5" x 3" x 1") weighs approximately eight ounces.
2. One bass fillet (8.75" long x 4.5" at widest point x 0.7" thickest point) weighs approximately eight ounces.
3. Three cod fillets (5" long x 2.5" at widest point x 1" at thickest point) weigh approximately eight ounces.
4. One cup of clam or seafood chowder weighs approximately eight to nine ounces.
5. One cup of seafood, crab or lobster salad weighs approximately eight ounces.
6. Five large shrimp (3 1/4" long as measured along the outer curvature) weigh approximately one ounce.
7. Two medium oysters weigh approximately one ounce.

Serving size--8 ounces:	Calories kcal	Carbo grams	Prot grams	Fat grams	Fat % of kcal	Chol mg
Albacore (tuna fish), unprepared	401	0	57.4	17.2	39	125
(tuna fish, canned in water)	288	0	63.5	1.8	6	143
Anchovy, unprepared	297	0	46.0	10.9	33	136
(clams, hard, raw)	111	9.5	14.7	0.9	7	113
Bluefish, baked/broiled	361	0	59.4	11.8	29	159
(fish, perch, baked/broiled)	265	0	56.4	2.7	10	261
Bluefish, fried	465	10.7	51.5	22.2	43	138
(bluefish, baked/broiled)	361	0	59.4	11.8	29	159
Bluefish, unprepared	281	0	45.4	9.5	30	134
(fish, haddock, unprepared)	197	0	42.9	1.6	7	129
Catfish, breaded fried	519	18.1	41.1	30.2	52	184
(fish, cod, unprepared)	186	0	40.3	1.6	8	97
Catfish, unprepared	215	0	37.2	6.3	28	131
(fish, haddock, unprepared)	197	0	42.9	1.6	7	129

( ) indicates possible substitute foods that are lower in calories and/or fat.

Serving size--8 ounces:	Calories kcal	Carbo grams	Prot grams	Fat grams	Fat % of kcal	Chol mg
Clam fritters	705	70.1	25.9	34.0	43	293
(clams, hard, raw)	111	9.5	14.7	0.9	7	113
Clams, breaded/fried	458	23.4	32.2	25.2	50	138
(clams, soft, unprepared)	122	4.5	19.5	2.3	17	113
Clams, canned	118	6.4	17.9	1.6	12	73
(clams, hard, raw)	111	9.5	14.7	0.9	7	113
Clams, hard, raw	111	9.5	14.7	0.9	7	113
(no alternate identified)						
Clams, soft, unprepared	122	4.5	19.5	2.3	17	113
(clams, hard, raw)	111	9.5	14.7	0.9	7	113
Crab, baked	333	8.8	59.4	4.8	13	383
(fish, cod, unprepared)	186	0	40.3	1.6	8	97
Crab cake	603	19.3	42.6	39.2	59	311
(crab, baked)	333	8.8	59.4	4.8	13	383
Crab, deviled	426	30.2	25.9	21.3	45	231
(steamed crab)	211	1.1	39.2	4.3	18	227
Crab imperial	333	8.8	33.1	17.2	46	318
(steamed crab)	211	1.1	39.2	4.3	18	227
Crab meat, canned	225	0	46.5	2.7	11	202
(clams, canned)	118	6.4	17.9	1.6	12	73
Crayfish	163	0	33.1	2.3	13	242
(clams, soft, unprepared)	122	4.5	19.5	2.3	17	113
Dogfish, spiny, unprepared	354	0	39.9	20.4	52	125
(fish, cod, unprepared)	186	0	40.3	1.6	8	97
Dolphin fish, unprepared	193	0	42.0	1.6	7	166
(fish, cod, unprepared)	186	0	40.3	1.6	8	97
Drum, red (redfish)	181	0	40.8	0.9	4	125
(clams, soft, unprepared)	122	4.5	19.5	2.3	17	113
Eel, american, unprepared	417	0	41.7	26.5	57	286
(fish, cod, unprepared)	186	0	40.3	1.6	8	97
Eel, smoked	748	0	42.2	63.1	76	145
(fish, smoked sturgeon)	392	0	70.8	10.0	23	181
Fish, alewife, unprepared	288	0	44.0	11.1	35	125
(fish, haddock, unprepared)	197	0	42.9	1.6	7	129

( ) indicates possible substitute foods that are lower in calories and/or fat.

Serving size--8 ounces:	Calories kcal	Carbo grams	Prot grams	Fat grams	Fat % of kcal	Chol mg
Fish, american shad, baked	456	0	52.6	25.6	51	156
(fish, american shad, creole)	345	3.6	34.0	19.7	51	100
Fish, american shad, creole	345	3.6	34.0	19.7	51	100
(shrimp creole)	159	10.7	25.4	1.4	8	188
Fish, american shad, unprepared	446	0	38.3	31.3	65	170
(fish, haddock, unprepared)	197	0	42.9	1.6	7	129
Fish, anchovy, pickled	399	0.7	43.5	23.4	53	125
(anchovy, unprepared)	297	0	46.0	10.9	33	136
Fish, barracuda, pacific, unprepared	256	0	47.6	5.9	21	125
(fish, cod, unprepared)	186	0	40.3	1.6	8	97
Fish, black bass, baked stuffed	587	25.9	36.7	35.8	55	104
(bluefish, baked/broiled)	361	0	59.4	11.8	29	159
Fish, black bullhead, unprepared	191	0	37.0	3.6	17	125
(fish, cod, unprepared)	186	0	40.3	1.6	8	97
Fish, black sea bass, unprepared	211	0	43.5	2.7	12	125
(fish, haddock, unprepared)	197	0	42.9	1.6	7	129
Fish, bluefin tuna, unprepared	327	0	52.8	11.1	31	86
(tuna fish, canned in water)	288	0	63.5	1.8	6	143
Fish, bonito, unprepared	381	0	54.4	16.6	39	125
(fish, grouper, unprepared)	209	0	44.0	2.3	10	84
Fish, brook trout, unprepared	229	0	43.5	4.8	19	111
(fish, haddock, unprepared)	197	0	42.9	1.6	7	129
Fish cakes, fried	390	21.1	33.3	18.1	42	95
(bluefish, baked/broiled)	361	0	59.4	11.8	29	159
Fish cakes, frozen, reheated	612	39.0	20.9	40.6	60	59
(bluefish, baked/broiled)	361	0	59.4	11.8	29	159
Fish, carp, unprepared	288	0	40.4	12.7	40	150
(fish, haddock, unprepared)	197	0	42.9	1.6	7	129
Fish chowder	177	12.9	13.4	7.9	40	35
(manhattan clam chowder)	73	11.3	2.0	2.0	25	2
Fish, cod, unprepared	186	0	40.3	1.6	8	97
(clams, soft, unprepared)	122	4.5	19.5	2.3	17	113
Fish, crappie, white	179	0	38.1	1.8	9	125
(clams, soft, unprepared)	122	4.5	19.5	2.3	17	113

( ) indicates possible substitute foods that are lower in calories and/or fat.

Serving size--8 ounces:	Calories kcal	Carbo grams	Prot grams	Fat grams	Fat % of kcal	Chol mg
Fish, creamed pollock, canned	290	9.1	31.5	13.4	42	84
(fish, cod, unprepared)	186	0	40.3	1.6	8	97
Fish, croacker, atlantic, baked	302	0	55.1	7.3	22	170
(fish, cod, unprepared)	186	0	40.3	1.6	8	97
Fish, croacker, atlantic, unprepared	236	0	40.4	7.3	28	138
(fish, croacker, white, unprepared)	191	0	40.8	1.8	8	125
Fish, croacker, white, unprepared	191	0	40.8	1.8	8	125
(fish, cod, unprepared)	186	0	40.3	1.6	8	97
Fish, drum, fresh-water, unprepared	270	0	39.7	11.1	37	145
(fish, cod, unprepared)	186	0	40.3	1.6	8	97
Fish, eulachon (smelt), unprepared	268	0	33.1	14.1	47	125
(fish, cod, unprepared)	186	0	40.3	1.6	8	97
Fish, flounder, baked	458	0	68.0	18.6	37	204
(fish, croacker, atlantic, baked)	302	0	55.1	7.3	22	170
Fish, gray and red snapper	211	0	44.9	2.0	9	125
(fish, cod, unprepared)	186	0	40.3	1.6	8	97
Fish, grouper, unprepared	209	0	44.0	2.3	10	84
(fish, cod, unprepared)	186	0	40.3	1.6	8	97
Fish, haddock, fried	374	13.2	44.5	14.5	35	145
(fish, haddock, smoked)	263	0	57.2	2.3	8	175
Fish, haddock, smoked	263	0	57.2	2.3	8	175
(fish, haddock, unprepared)	197	0	42.9	1.6	7	129
Fish, haddock, unprepared	197	0	42.9	1.6	7	129
(fish, hake/whiting, unprepared)	168	0	37.4	0.9	5	125
Fish, hake/whiting, unprepared	168	0	37.4	0.9	5	125
(clams, soft, unprepared)	122	4.5	19.5	2.3	17	113
Fish, halibut, california	220	0	44.9	3.2	13	113
(fish, haddock, unprepared)	197	0	42.9	1.6	7	129
Fish, halibut, greenland, unprepared	422	0	32.7	31.3	67	104
(fish, halibut, california)	220	0	44.9	3.2	13	113
Fish, herring/tomato sauce, canned	399	8.4	35.8	23.8	54	177
(tuna fish, canned in water)	288	0	63.5	1.8	6	143
Fish, herring, atlantic, unprepared	358	0	40.8	20.4	51	136
(fish, cod, unprepared)	186	0	40.3	1.6	8	97

( ) indicates possible substitute foods that are lower in calories and/or fat.

Serving size--8 ounces:	Calories kcal	Carbo grams	Prot grams	Fat grams	Fat % of kcal	Chol mg
Fish, herring, pacific, unprepared	442	0	37.2	31.5	64	175
(fish, cod, unprepared)	186	0	40.3	1.6	8	97
Fish, herring, pickled	594	21.8	32.2	40.8	62	29
(fish, anchovy, pickled)	399	0.7	43.5	23.4	53	125
Fish, herring, plain, canned	472	0	45.1	30.8	59	220
(tuna fish, canned in water)	288	0	63.5	1.8	6	143
Fish, herring, smoked, hard	680	0	83.7	35.8	47	411
(fish, smoked sturgeon)	392	0	70.8	10.0	23	181
Fish, jack mackerel, unprepared	356	0	45.6	17.9	45	107
(fish, cod, unprepared)	186	0	40.3	1.6	8	97
Fish, lake trout, unprepared	381	0	41.5	22.7	54	125
(fish, haddock, unprepared)	197	0	42.9	1.6	7	129
Fish, mackerel, atlantic, broiled	594	0	54.0	40.4	61	170
(bluefish, baked/broiled)	361	0	59.4	11.8	29	159
Fish, mackerel, atlantic, canned	415	0	43.8	25.2	55	213
(tuna fish, canned in water)	288	0	63.5	1.8	6	143
Fish, mackerel, pacific, canned	408	0	47.9	22.7	50	213
(tuna fish, canned in water)	288	0	63.5	1.8	6	143
Fish, mackerel, salted	692	0	42.0	56.9	74	215
(fish, mackerel, pacific, canned)	408	0	47.9	22.7	50	213
Fish, mackerel, smoked	497	0	54.0	29.5	53	215
(fish, mackerel, pacific, canned)	408	0	47.9	22.7	50	213
Fish, mullet, striped, unprepared	265	0	43.8	8.6	29	111
(fish, cod, unprepared)	186	0	40.3	1.6	8	97
Fish, orange roughy, unprepared	286	0	33.3	15.9	50	45
(fish, cod, unprepared)	186	0	40.3	1.6	8	97
Fish, perch, baked/broiled	265	0	56.4	2.7	10	261
(fish, cod, unprepared)	186	0	40.3	1.6	8	97
Fish, perch, fried	515	15.4	43.1	30.2	53	132
(bluefish, baked/broiled)	361	0	59.4	11.8	29	159
Fish, perch, unprepared	206	0	44.2	2.0	9	204
(fish, cod, unprepared)	186	0	40.3	1.6	8	97
Fish, pickerel (pike), chain	191	0	42.4	1.1	5	125
(fish, cod, unprepared)	186	0	40.3	1.6	8	97

( ) indicates possible substitute foods that are lower in calories and/or fat.

Serving size--8 ounces:	Calories kcal	Carbo grams	Prot grams	Fat grams	Fat % of kcal	Chol mg
Fish, pike, blue, unprepared	204	0	43.3	2.0	9	125
(fish, cod, unprepared)	186	0	40.3	1.6	8	97
Fish, pike, northern, unprepared	200	0	43.8	1.6	7	88
(fish, cod, unprepared)	186	0	40.3	1.6	8	97
Fish, pike, walleye, unprepared	211	0	43.3	2.7	12	195
(fish, pickerel (pike), chain)	191	0	42.4	1.1	5	125
Fish, pollock, unprepared	209	0	44.0	2.3	10	161
(fish, cod, unprepared)	186	0	40.3	1.6	8	97
Fish, porgy/scup, unprepared	238	0	42.8	6.1	24	118
(fish, cod, unprepared)	186	0	40.3	1.6	8	97
Fish, rainbow trout, canned	474	0	46.7	30.4	58	120
(tuna fish, canned in water)	288	0	63.5	1.8	6	143
Fish, rainbow trout, unprepared	268	0	46.5	7.7	26	129
(fish, brook trout, unprepared)	229	0	43.5	4.8	19	111
Fish, salmon, atlantic, canned	460	0	49.2	27.7	54	84
(fish, cod, unprepared)	186	0	40.3	1.6	8	97
Fish, salmon, broiled or baked	413	0	61.2	16.8	37	107
(fish, cod, unprepared)	186	0	40.3	1.6	8	97
Fish, salmon, chinook, canned	476	0	44.5	31.8	60	77
(fish, cod, unprepared)	186	0	40.3	1.6	8	97
Fish, salmon, coho, canned	347	0	47.2	16.1	42	82
(tuna fish, canned in water)	288	0	63.5	1.8	6	143
Fish, salmon, pink, canned	315	0	44.9	13.6	39	125
(tuna fish, canned in water)	288	0	63.5	1.8	6	143
Fish, salmon, sockeye, canned	347	0	46.5	16.6	43	100
(fish, cod, unprepared)	186	0	40.3	1.6	8	97
Fish, sardines, canned in oil	472	1.4	55.8	25.9	49	322
(fish, sardines, canned in water)	445	3.9	42.6	27.2	55	249
Fish, sardines, canned in water	445	3.9	42.6	27.2	55	249
(tuna fish, canned in water)	288	0	63.5	1.8	6	143
Fish, sardines in tomato sauce	404	0	37.0	27.2	61	138
(tuna fish, canned in water)	288	0	63.5	1.8	6	143
Fish, sea bass, white, unprepared	220	0	41.7	4.5	18	93
(fish, cod, unprepared)	186	0	40.3	1.6	8	97

( ) indicates possible substitute foods that are lower in calories and/or fat.

Serving size--8 ounces:	Calories kcal	Carbo grams	Prot grams	Fat grams	Fat % of kcal	Chol mg
Fish, small and large mouth bass	258	0	42.9	8.4	31	154
(fish, sea bass, white, unprepared)	220	0	41.7	4.5	18	93
Fish, smelt, atlantic, canned	454	0	41.7	30.6	61	122
(tuna fish, canned in water)	288	0	63.5	1.8	6	143
Fish, smelt, atlantic, unprepared	222	0	42.2	4.8	19	125
(fish, cod, unprepared)	186	0	40.3	1.6	8	97
Fish, smoked herring, kipper	479	0	50.3	29.3	55	247
(fish, smoked sturgeon)	392	0	70.8	10.0	23	181
Fish, smoked salmon (lox)	265	0	41.5	9.8	33	52
(fish, cod, unprepared)	186	0	40.3	1.6	8	97
Fish, smoked sturgeon	392	0	70.8	10.0	23	181
(fish, sturgeon, unprepared)	238	0	36.5	9.1	36	136
Fish, spot, baked	669	0	51.7	49.7	67	161
(bluefish, baked/broiled)	361	0	59.4	11.8	29	159
Fish sticks, frozen, cooked	617	54.0	35.4	27.7	40	254
(bluefish, baked/broiled)	361	0	59.4	11.8	29	159
Fish, striped bass, oven-fried	445	15.2	48.8	19.3	39	143
(bluefish, baked/broiled)	361	0	59.4	11.8	29	159
Fish, striped bass, unprepared	220	0	40.1	5.2	21	181
(fish, cod, unprepared)	186	0	40.3	1.6	8	97
Fish, sturgeon, unprepared	238	0	36.5	9.1	36	136
(fish, cod, unprepared)	186	0	40.3	1.6	8	97
Fish, sucker, carp, unprepared	209	0	38.1	5.2	22	93
(fish, cod, unprepared)	186	0	40.3	1.6	8	97
Fish, tautog, unprepared	202	0	42.2	2.5	11	125
(fish, cod, unprepared)	186	0	40.3	1.6	8	97
Fish, terripin, unprepared	252	0	42.2	7.9	28	113
(fish, cod, unprepared)	186	0	40.3	1.6	8	97
Fish, tomcod, atlantic, unprepared	175	0	39.0	0.9	5	125
(clams, soft, unprepared)	122	4.5	19.5	2.3	17	113
Fish, turbot, fried	374	0	83.9	14.5	35	265
(fish, cod, unprepared)	186	0	40.3	1.6	8	97
Fish, turbot, unprepared	215	0	36.3	6.6	28	109
(fish, cod, unprepared)	186	0	40.3	1.6	8	97

( ) indicates possible substitute foods that are lower in calories and/or fat.

Serving size--8 ounces:	Calories kcal	Carbo grams	Prot grams	Fat grams	Fat % of kcal	Chol mg
Fish, white bass, steamed	222	0	40.8	5.2	21	125
(fish, cod, unprepared)	186	0	40.3	1.6	8	97
Fish, yellowfin tuna, unprepared	245	0	53.1	2.0	7	102
(fish, cod, unprepared)	186	0	40.3	1.6	8	97
Fish, yellowtail, pacific	331	0	52.4	11.8	32	125
(fish, cod, unprepared)	186	0	40.3	1.6	8	97
Flatfishes (sole), unprepared	206	0	42.6	2.7	12	109
(fish, cod, unprepared)	186	0	40.3	1.6	8	97
French-fried shrimp	510	22.7	46.0	24.5	43	340
(shrimp, steamed/boiled)	224	0	47.4	2.5	11	442
Kingfish, unprepared	238	0	41.5	6.8	26	125
(fish, cod, unprepared)	186	0	40.3	1.6	8	97
Lobster newburg	440	11.6	42.0	24.0	49	413
(lobster, spiny)	254	5.4	46.7	3.4	13	159
Lobster, northern	204	1.1	42.6	2.0	9	215
(crayfish)	163	0	33.5	2.3	13	242
Lobster salad	249	5.2	22.9	14.5	52	104
(shrimp cocktail)	216	35.6	17.0	1.2	5	118
Lobster, spiny	254	5.4	46.7	3.4	13	159
(clams, soft, unprepared)	122	4.5	19.5	2.3	17	113
Manhattan clam chowder	73	11.3	2.0	2.0	25	2
(crab ready-to-serve soup)	70	9.5	5.2	1.4	18	9
Mussels, canned	259	3.4	41.3	7.5	26	102
(mussels, steamed)	195	8.4	27.0	5.0	23	64
Mussels, steamed	195	8.4	27.0	5.0	23	64
(clams, hard, raw)	111	9.5	14.7	0.9	7	113
New england clam chowder	150	15.2	8.6	6.1	37	20
(manhattan clam chowder)	73	11.3	2.0	2.0	25	2
Octopus	186	5.0	33.8	2.3	11	109
(clams, hard, raw)	111	9.5	14.7	0.9	7	113
Oyster stew, prepared	220	10.2	11.8	14.5	59	82
(manhattan clam chowder)	73	11.3	2.0	2.0	25	2
Oysters, atlantic, raw	156	8.8	16.1	5.7	33	120
(clams, hard, raw)	111	9.5	14.7	0.9	7	113

( ) indicates possible substitute foods that are lower in calories and/or fat.

Serving size--8 ounces:	Calories kcal	Carbo grams	Prot grams	Fat grams	Fat % of kcal	Chol mg
Oysters, fried	446	26.3	19.9	28.6	58	184
(oysters, atlantic, raw)	156	8.8	16.1	5.7	33	120
Oysters, pacific, raw	184	11.1	21.3	5.2	25	113
(clams, hard, raw)	111	9.5	14.7	0.9	7	113
Sablefish, unprepared	442	0	30.4	34.7	71	111
(fish, cod, unprepared)	186	0	40.3	1.6	8	97
Salmon rice loaf	277	16.6	27.2	10.2	33	48
(shrimp creole)	159	10.7	25.4	1.4	8	188
Scallops, fried	488	22.9	41.1	24.7	46	138
(scallops, unprepared)	254	7.5	52.6	3.2	11	120
Scallops, unprepared	254	7.5	52.6	3.2	11	120
(clams, hard, raw)	111	9.5	14.7	0.9	7	113
Seaweed, agar, fresh	59	15.4	1.1	0	0	0
(watercress)	24	3.0	5.2	0.2	14	0
Seaweed, irish moss, fresh	111	27.9	3.4	0.5	4	0
(seaweed, agar, fresh)	59	15.4	1.1	0	0	0
Seaweed, kelp, fresh	98	21.8	3.9	1.4	13	0
(seaweed, agar, fresh)	59	15.4	1.1	0	0	0
Seaweed, laver, fresh	79	11.6	13.2	0.7	8	0
(seaweed, agar, fresh)	59	15.4	1.1	0	0	0
Seaweed, spirulina, fresh	59	5.4	13.4	0.9	14	0
(watercress)	24	3.0	5.2	0.2	14	0
Seaweed, wakame, fresh	102	20.6	6.8	1.4	12	0
(seaweed, agar, fresh)	59	15.4	1.1	0	0	0
Shellfish, abalone, canned	181	5.2	36.3	0.7	3	107
(clams, hard, raw)	111	9.5	14.7	0.9	7	113
Shellfish, abalone, unprepared	238	13.6	38.8	1.8	7	193
(clams, hard, raw)	111	9.5	14.7	0.9	7	113
Shrimp cocktail	215	35.6	17.0	1.1	5	118
(crayfish)	163	0	33.5	2.3	13	242
Shrimp, frozen, breaded, unprep.	315	45.1	27.9	1.6	5	231
(crayfish)	163	0	33.5	2.3	13	242
Shrimp or lobster paste	408	3.4	47.2	21.3	47	390
(lobster, spiny)	254	5.4	46.7	3.4	13	159

( ) indicates possible substitute foods that are lower in calories and/or fat.

Serving size--8 ounces:	Calories kcal	Carbo grams	Prot grams	Fat grams	Fat % of kcal	Chol mg
Shrimp salad	358	5.2	24.0	26.5	67	212
(shrimp cocktail)	215	35.6	17.0	1.1	5	118
Shrimp, steamed/boiled	224	0	47.4	2.5	11	442
(crayfish)	163	0	33.5	2.3	13	242
Skate (raja fish), unprepared	222	0	48.8	1.6	6	125
(fish, cod, unprepared)	186	0	40.3	1.6	8	97
Snail (escargot), unprepared	204	4.5	36.5	3.2	14	113
(clams, soft, unprepared)	122	4.5	19.5	2.3	17	113
Snapper, baked/broiled	290	0	59.6	3.9	12	107
(fish, cod, unprepared)	186	0	40.3	1.6	8	97
Squid	209	7.0	35.4	3.2	14	528
(octopus)	186	5.0	33.8	2.3	11	109
Steamed crab	211	1.1	39.2	4.3	18	227
(clams, soft, unprepared)	122	4.5	19.5	2.3	17	113
Sturgeon caviar	594	7.5	61.0	34.0	53	680
(shrimp or lobster paste)	408	3.4	47.2	21.3	47	390
Swordfish, broiled	352	0	57.6	11.6	30	113
(fish, cod, unprepared)	186	0	40.3	1.6	8	97
Tilefish, baked	333	0	55.6	10.7	29	145
(fish, cod, unprepared)	186	0	40.3	1.6	8	97
Trout, baked/broiled	342	0	59.0	9.8	26	166
(fish, cod, unprepared)	186	0	40.3	1.6	8	97
Tuna fish, canned in oil	653	0	54.9	46.5	64	125
(tuna fish, canned in water)	288	0	63.5	1.8	6	143
Tuna fish, canned in water	288	0	63.5	1.8	6	143
(fish, cod, unprepared)	186	0	40.3	1.6	8	97
Tuna salad	424	21.3	36.3	21.1	45	29
(tuna fish, canned in water)	288	0	63.5	1.8	6	143
Turtle, green, unprepared	202	0	44.9	1.1	5	113
(fish, cod, unprepared)	186	0	40.3	1.6	8	97
Whitefish, lake, unprepared	304	0	43.3	13.4	40	136
(fish, cod, unprepared)	186	0	40.3	1.6	8	97
Whitefish, smoked	245	0	53.1	2.0	7	75
(fish, cod, unprepared)	186	0	40.3	1.6	8	97

( ) indicates possible substitute foods that are lower in calories and/or fat.

Serving size--8 ounces:	Calories kcal	Carbo grams	Prot grams	Fat grams	Fat % of kcal	Chol mg
Whitefish, stuffed, baked	488	13.2	34.5	31.8	59	100
(whitefish, smoked)	245	0	53.1	2.0	7	75
Wreckfish, unprepared	259	0	41.7	8.8	31	125
(fish, cod, unprepared)	186	0	40.3	1.6	8	97

( ) indicates possible substitute foods that are lower in calories and/or fat.

SOUP

The serving size used for this category is 8 ounces. To facilitate comparisons among canned condensed soups versus commercial ready-to-serve soups versus dehydrated soups, all the information is presented as prepared soup. Unless otherwise indicated, all soups are canned condensed soups prepared with water. Any food item that contains the designation "w/milk" is a condensed soup prepared with milk. Homemade soups may vary significantly from commercial soups; for a more accurate representation of the nutritional content of a homemade soup, analyze its specific ingredients.

Weights and Measures

1. One cup (8 fluid ounces) of soup weighs approximately eight to nine ounces.
2. One can of condensed soup (10.5 ounce can) yields approximately 2 1/2 cups of prepared soup.

Serving size--8 ounces:	Calories kcal	Carbo grams	Prot grams	Fat grams	Fat % of kcal	Chol mg
Bean with bacon soup	145	19.3	6.8	5.0	31	2
(tomato soup)	77	15.0	1.8	1.8	21	0
Bean with ham chunky soup	215	25.4	11.8	7.9	33	20
(tomato soup)	77	15.0	1.8	1.8	21	0
Beef broth ready-to-serve soup	16	0	2.5	0.5	28	0
(dehydrated beef bouillon prepared)	7	0.7	0.5	0.2	26	0
Beef chunky soup	161	18.4	11.1	4.8	27	14
(beef noodle soup)	77	8.2	4.3	2.9	34	5
Beef mushroom soup	70	5.9	5.2	2.7	35	6
(chicken gumbo soup)	52	7.7	2.5	1.4	24	3
Beef noodle soup	77	8.2	4.3	2.9	34	5
(chicken noodle soup)	70	8.6	3.6	2.0	26	6
Beef stew	202	14.1	14.5	9.8	44	59
(vegetable chunky ready serve soup)	116	17.9	3.4	3.4	26	0
Black bean soup	104	17.5	5.4	1.6	14	0
(chicken gumbo soup)	52	7.7	2.5	1.4	24	3

( ) indicates possible substitute foods that are lower in calories and/or fat.

Serving size--8 ounces:	Calories kcal	Carbo grams	Prot grams	Fat grams	Fat % of kcal	Chol mg
Cheese soup	138	9.3	4.8	9.3	61	26
(tomato soup)	77	15.0	1.8	1.8	21	0
Cheese soup w/milk	209	14.7	8.6	13.2	57	43
(tomato soup w/milk)	147	20.4	5.7	5.4	33	16
Chicken bouillon prepared	7	0.5	0.5	0.5	64	0
(dehydrated beef bouillon prepared)	7	0.7	0.5	0.2	26	0
Chicken broth soup	36	0.9	5.0	1.1	27	1
(chicken bouillon prepared)	7	0.5	0.5	0.5	64	0
Chicken chunky soup	161	15.6	11.6	5.9	33	27
(chicken gumbo soup)	52	7.7	2.5	1.4	24	3
Chicken gumbo soup	52	7.7	2.5	1.4	24	3
(chicken broth soup)	36	0.9	5.0	1.1	27	1
Chicken noodle chunky soup	166	16.1	12.0	5.7	31	18
(chicken gumbo soup)	52	7.7	2.5	1.4	24	3
Chicken noodle soup	70	8.6	3.6	2.0	26	6
(chicken gumbo soup)	52	7.7	2.5	1.4	24	3
Chicken vegetable chunky soup	156	17.9	11.6	4.5	26	16
(chicken gumbo soup)	52	7.7	2.5	1.4	24	3
Chicken vegetable soup	70	8.2	3.4	2.3	34	9
(chicken gumbo soup)	52	7.7	2.5	1.4	24	3
Chicken with rice chunky soup	120	12.2	11.6	2.9	22	11
(chicken gumbo soup)	52	7.7	2.5	1.4	24	3
Chicken with rice soup	57	6.6	3.4	1.8	28	6
(chicken gumbo soup)	52	7.7	2.5	1.4	24	3
Chili beef soup	147	18.6	5.9	5.7	35	11
(tomato soup)	77	15.0	1.8	1.8	21	0
Consomme with gel	27	1.6	5.0	0	0	0
(dehydrated beef bouillon prepared)	7	0.7	0.5	0.2	26	0
Crab ready-to-serve soup	70	9.5	5.2	1.4	18	9
(chicken gumbo soup)	52	7.7	2.5	1.4	24	3
Cream of asparagus soup	79	9.8	2.0	3.9	44	5
(chicken gumbo soup)	52	7.7	2.5	1.4	24	3
Cream of chicken soup	107	8.4	3.2	6.8	57	9
(tomato soup)	77	15.0	1.8	1.8	21	0

( ) indicates possible substitute foods that are lower in calories and/or fat.

Serving size--8 ounces:	Calories kcal	Carbo grams	Prot grams	Fat grams	Fat % of kcal	Chol mg
Cream of mushroom soup	118	8.4	1.8	8.6	66	1
(tomato soup)	77	15.0	1.8	1.8	21	0
Cream of potato soup	68	10.4	1.6	2.3	30	6
(chicken gumbo soup)	52	7.7	2.5	1.4	24	3
Dehydrated beef bouillon prepared	7	0.7	0.5	0.2	26	0
(no alternate identified)						
Escarole ready-to-serve soup	25	1.6	1.4	1.6	58	2
(dehydrated beef bouillon prepared)	7	0.7	0.5	0.2	26	0
Fish chowder	177	12.9	13.4	7.9	40	35
(crab ready-to-serve soup)	70	9.5	5.2	1.4	18	9
Gazpacho ready-to-serve soup	52	0.7	8.2	2.0	35	0
(escarole ready-to-serve soup)	25	1.6	1.4	1.6	58	2
Lentil w/ham ready-to-serve soup	127	18.6	8.4	2.5	18	7
(gazpacho ready-to-serve soup)	52	0.7	8.2	2.0	35	0
Manhattan clam chowder	73	11.3	2.0	2.0	25	2
(chicken gumbo soup)	52	7.7	2.5	1.4	24	3
Manhattan clam chowder chunky soup	127	17.7	6.8	3.2	23	14
(crab ready-to-serve soup)	70	9.5	5.2	1.4	18	9
Minestrone chunky soup	120	19.5	4.8	2.7	20	5
(chicken gumbo soup)	52	7.7	2.5	1.4	24	3
Minestrone soup	77	10.4	4.1	2.3	27	1
(chicken gumbo soup)	52	7.7	2.5	1.4	24	3
New england clam chowder	150	15.2	8.6	6.1	37	20
(manhattan clam chowder)	73	11.3	2.0	2.0	25	2
Onion soup	52	7.7	3.6	1.6	28	0
(dehydrated beef bouillon prepared)	7	0.7	0.5	0.2	26	0
Oyster stew	125	9.1	5.7	7.3	53	29
(crab ready-to-serve soup)	70	9.5	5.2	1.4	18	9
Pea green soup	143	22.9	7.5	2.5	16	0
(tomato soup)	77	15.0	1.8	1.8	21	0
Pepper pot soup	95	8.8	5.9	4.3	41	9
(chicken gumbo soup)	52	7.7	2.5	1.4	24	3
Split pea with ham chunky soup	175	25.4	10.4	3.9	20	7
(chicken gumbo soup)	52	7.7	2.5	1.4	24	3

( ) indicates possible substitute foods that are lower in calories and/or fat.

Serving size--8 ounces:	Calories kcal	Carbo grams	Prot grams	Fat grams	Fat % of kcal	Chol mg
Tomato bisque soup	109	21.1	2.0	2.3	19	5
(tomato soup)	77	15.0	1.8	1.8	21	0
Tomato soup	77	15.0	1.8	1.8	21	0
(gazpacho ready-to-serve soup)	52	0.7	8.2	2.0	35	0
Tomato soup w/milk	147	20.4	5.7	5.4	33	16
(tomato soup)	77	15.0	1.8	1.8	21	0
Tomato with rice soup	107	19.5	1.8	2.5	21	1
(tomato soup)	77	15.0	1.8	1.8	21	0
Turkey chunky ready-to-serve soup	129	13.6	9.8	4.3	30	9
(turkey noodle soup)	64	7.9	3.6	1.8	25	5
Turkey noodle soup	64	7.9	3.6	1.8	25	5
(chicken gumbo soup)	52	7.7	2.5	1.4	24	3
Turkey vegetable soup	68	7.9	2.9	2.9	38	1
(chicken gumbo soup)	52	7.7	2.5	1.4	24	3
Vegetable beef soup	73	9.3	5.0	1.8	22	5
(turkey vegetable soup)	68	7.9	2.9	2.9	38	1
Vegetable chunky ready serve soup	116	17.9	3.4	3.4	26	0
(turkey vegetable soup)	68	7.9	2.9	2.9	38	1
Vegetarian vegetable soup	68	11.1	2.0	1.8	24	0
(gazpacho ready-to-serve soup)	52	0.7	8.2	2.0	35	0

( ) indicates possible substitute foods that are lower in calories and/or fat.

SYRUPS, JAMS AND PRESERVES

Syrups, jams and preserves are listed in this category with a serving size of 0.5 ounces, an amount roughly equivalent to 1 tablespoon or 3 teaspoons.

Serving size--0.5 ounce:	Calories kcal	Carbo grams	Prot grams	Fat grams	Fat % of kcal	Chol mg
Apple butter	26	6.6	0.1	0.1	3	0
(low-calorie syrup)	11	3.0	0	0	0	0
Apple jelly	39	10.0	0	0	0	0
(apple butter)	26	6.6	0.1	0.1	3	0
Apricot jam	39	9.9	0.1	0	0	0
(low-calorie imitation jelly)	24	6.0	0	0	0	0
Apricot jelly	39	10.0	0	0	0	0
(low-calorie imitation jelly)	24	6.0	0	0	0	0
Apricot preserves	39	9.9	0.1	0	0	0
(low-calorie imitation jelly)	24	6.0	0	0	0	0
Artificial sweetener	0	0	0	0	0	0
(no alternate identified)						
Black raspberry jam	39	9.9	0.1	0	0	0
(low-calorie imitation jelly)	24	6.0	0	0	0	0
Black raspberry jelly	39	10.0	0	0	0	0
(low-calorie imitation jelly)	24	6.0	0	0	0	0
Blackberry jam	39	9.9	0.1	0	0	0
(low-calorie imitation jelly)	24	6.0	0	0	0	0
Blackberry jelly	39	10.0	0	0	0	0
(low-calorie imitation jelly)	24	6.0	0	0	0	0
Boysenberry jam	39	9.9	0.1	0	0	0
(low-calorie imitation jelly)	24	6.0	0	0	0	0
Cane syrup	37	9.6	0	0	0	0
(low-calorie syrup)	11	3.0	0	0	0	0
Cherry jam	39	9.9	0.1	0	0	0
(low-calorie imitation jelly)	24	6.0	0	0	0	0
Cherry jelly	39	10.0	0	0	0	0
(low-calorie imitation jelly)	24	6.0	0	0	0	0

( ) indicates possible substitute foods that are lower in calories and/or fat.

Serving size--0.5 ounce:	Calories kcal	Carbo grams	Prot grams	Fat grams	Fat % of kcal	Chol mg
Chocolate syrup, fudge type	47	7.7	0.7	1.9	36	0
(chocolate syrup, thin type)	35	8.9	0.3	0.3	8	0
Chocolate syrup, thin type	35	8.9	0.3	0.3	8	0
(low-calorie syrup)	11	3.0	0	0	0	0
Corn syrup, light and dark	41	10.6	0	0	0	0
(maple syrup)	36	9.2	0	0	0	0
Elderberry jelly	39	10.0	0	0	0	0
(low-calorie imitation jelly)	24	6.0	0	0	0	0
Grape jam	39	9.9	0.1	0	0	0
(low-calorie imitation jelly)	24	6.0	0	0	0	0
Grape jelly	39	10.0	0	0	0	0
(low-calorie imitation jelly)	24	6.0	0	0	0	0
Honey	43	11.7	0	0	0	0
(low-calorie syrup)	11	3.0	0	0	0	0
Maple syrup	36	9.2	0	0	0	0
(low-calorie syrup)	11	3.0	0	0	0	0
Marmalade, citrus	36	9.9	0.1	0	0	0
(low-calorie imitation jelly)	24	6.0	0	0	0	0
Mint flavor apple jelly	39	10.0	0	0	0	0
(apple butter)	26	6.6	0.1	0.1	3	0
Molasses, cane, light	36	9.2	0	0	0	0
(molasses, cane, medium)	33	8.5	0	0	0	0
Molasses, cane, medium	33	8.5	0	0	0	0
(low-calorie syrup)	11	3.0	0	0	0	0
Orange marmalade	36	9.9	0.1	0	0	0
(low-calorie imitation jelly)	24	6.0	0	0	0	0
Peach preserves	39	9.9	0.1	0	0	0
(low-calorie imitation jelly)	24	6.0	0	0	0	0
Pineapple preserves	39	9.9	0.1	0	0	0
(low-calorie imitation jelly)	24	6.0	0	0	0	0
Red raspberry jam	39	9.9	0.1	0	0	0
(low-calorie imitation jelly)	24	6.0	0	0	0	0
Red raspberry jelly	39	10.0	0	0	0	0
(low-calorie imitation jelly)	24	6.0	0	0	0	0

( ) indicates possible substitute foods that are lower in calories and/or fat.

Serving size--0.5 ounce:	Calories kcal	Carbo grams	Prot grams	Fat grams	Fat % of kcal	Chol mg
Sorghum syrup	41	10.6	0	0	0	0
(low-calorie syrup)	11	3.0	0	0	0	0
Strawberry jam	39	9.9	0.1	0	0	0
(low-calorie imitation jelly)	24	6.0	0	0	0	0
Strawberry jelly	39	10.0	0	0	0	0
(low-calorie imitation jelly)	24	6.0	0	0	0	0
Strawberry preserves	39	9.9	0.1	0	0	0
(low-calorie imitation jelly)	24	6.0	0	0	0	0

( ) indicates possible substitute foods that are lower in calories and/or fat.

VEGETABLES AND SALADS

The serving size used for this category is the same as for the Fruit and Juice category: 4 ounces. Please note that for canned vegetables the weight, and therefore the nutritional values, include the liquid used in canning. It is therefore more meaningful to compare two types of canned vegetables rather than one that is canned and another vegetable that is not.

Weights and Measures

1. One cup of coleslaw, potato salad, or egg salad weighs approximately four ounces.
2. One eight-inch stalk of celery weighs approximately one and a half ounces.
3. One 2 1/4" diameter potato weighs approximately four ounces.
4. One 2.5" diameter tomato weighs approximately four ounces.
5. One cup of chopped mushrooms weighs approximately two and a half ounces.
6. One cup of mixed vegetables (frozen or fresh) after cooking weighs approximately five to six ounces.

Serving size--4 ounces:	Calories kcal	Carbo grams	Prot grams	Fat grams	Fat % of kcal	Chol mg
Alfalfa	33	4.3	4.5	0.8	22	0
(spinach, fresh)	25	4.0	3.3	0.3	11	0
Amaranth	29	4.5	2.8	0.3	9	0
(iceberg lettuce)	15	2.4	1.1	0.2	12	0
Arrowhead	112	22.9	6.0	0.3	2	0
(asparagus, fresh)	25	4.2	3.5	0.2	7	0
Artichokes, fresh	53	11.9	3.7	0.1	1	0
(asparagus, fresh)	26	5.1	2.6	0.2	6	0
Asparagus, canned	16	2.6	2.0	0.2	11	0
(squash, zucchini)	16	3.3	1.4	0.1	6	0
Asparagus, fresh	26	5.1	2.6	0.2	6	0
(squash, zucchini)	16	3.3	1.4	0.1	6	0
Avocado (guacamole dip)	189	7.1	2.4	18.6	89	0
(mexican salsa)	24	5.6	0.8	0	0	0

( ) indicates possible substitute foods that are lower in calories and/or fat.

Serving size--4 ounces:	Calories kcal	Carbo grams	Prot grams	Fat grams	Fat % of kcal	Chol mg
Baked beans (without pork) canned	105	23.2	5.4	0.5	4	0
(navy beans, canned)	76	14.7	6.9	0.8	9	0
Balsam-pear leaf	34	3.7	6.0	0.8	21	0
(spinach, fresh)	25	4.0	3.3	0.3	11	0
Bamboo shoots, canned	22	3.6	1.9	0.5	20	0
(taro shoots)	12	2.6	1.0	0.1	7	0
Bamboo shoots, fresh	31	5.9	2.9	0.3	9	0
(taro shoots)	12	2.6	1.0	0.1	7	0
Beans, dry, white, raw	377	68.3	26.5	0.9	2	0
(navy beans, canned)	76	14.7	6.9	0.8	9	0
Beans and franks, canned	161	17.5	7.7	7.5	40	7
(baked beans (without pork) canned)	105	23.2	5.4	0.5	4	0
Beans, dry, red, raw	389	70.2	25.5	1.7	4	0
(navy beans, canned)	76	14.7	6.9	0.8	9	0
Beet greens, fresh	22	4.5	2.0	0.1	4	0
(watercress)	12	1.5	2.6	0.1	7	0
Beets, canned	33	7.7	0.9	0.1	3	0
(green beans (string beans), canned)	17	4.0	0.9	0.1	5	0
Beets, fresh	50	11.3	1.7	0.1	2	0
(beet greens, fresh)	22	4.5	2.0	0.1	4	0
Borage	24	3.5	2.0	0.8	30	0
(watercress)	12	1.5	2.6	0.1	7	0
Broccoli, fresh	32	5.9	3.4	0.3	8	0
(asparagus, fresh)	26	5.1	2.6	0.2	6	0
Brussels sprouts, fresh	49	10.2	3.9	0.3	6	0
(broccoli, fresh)	32	5.9	3.4	0.3	8	0
Burdock root	82	19.6	1.7	0.1	1	0
(beets, fresh)	50	11.3	1.7	0.1	2	0
Butterbur, fresh	16	4.1	0.5	0	0	0
(watercress)	12	1.5	2.6	0.1	7	0
Cabbage, boiled	24	5.4	1.1	0.3	11	0
(pak-choi cabbage, fresh)	15	2.5	1.7	0.2	12	0
Cabbage, fresh	27	6.1	1.4	0.2	7	0
(pak-choi cabbage, fresh)	15	2.5	1.7	0.2	12	0

( ) indicates possible substitute foods that are lower in calories and/or fat.

Serving size--4 ounces:	Calories kcal	Carbo grams	Prot grams	Fat grams	Fat % of kcal	Chol mg
Carrot juice	45	10.5	1.0	0.1	2	0
(tomato juice)	19	4.8	0.9	0.1	5	0
Carrot salad	205	38.4	2.0	6.7	29	5
(carrots, fresh)	49	11.5	1.1	0.2	4	0
Carrots, canned	26	5.8	0.7	0.2	7	0
(green beans (string beans), canned)	17	4.0	0.9	0.1	5	0
Carrots, fresh	49	11.5	1.1	0.2	4	0
(turnips, fresh)	31	7.0	1.0	0.1	3	0
Cassava	136	30.5	3.5	0.5	3	0
(potatoes, boiled)	99	22.8	2.2	0.1	1	0
Cauliflower	27	5.6	2.3	0.2	7	0
(cucumber)	15	3.3	0.6	0.1	6	0
Celeriac	44	10.4	1.7	0.3	6	0
(celery)	18	4.1	0.8	0.1	5	0
Celery	18	4.1	0.8	0.1	5	0
(cucumber)	15	3.3	0.6	0.1	6	0
Chayote fruit	27	6.1	1.0	0.3	10	0
(squash, zucchini)	16	3.3	1.4	0.1	6	0
Chicken salad	395	0.9	23.2	32.9	75	91
(chicken breast, meat only, roasted)	187	0	35.2	4.1	20	96
Chickpeas, canned	135	25.6	5.6	1.2	8	0
(navy beans, canned)	76	14.7	6.9	0.8	9	0
Chicory greens	26	5.3	1.9	0.3	10	0
(iceberg lettuce)	15	2.4	1.1	0.2	12	0
Chicory roots	83	19.8	1.6	0.2	2	0
(beets, fresh)	50	11.3	1.7	0.1	2	0
Chives, fresh	34	4.9	3.7	0.8	17	0
(no alternate identified)						
Coleslaw	78	14.1	1.5	2.9	33	9
(garden salad (without dressing))	17	3.2	1.1	0.2	11	0
Collards	35	8.0	1.8	0.2	4	0
(watercress)	12	1.5	2.6	0.1	7	0
Corn, creamed, canned	82	20.5	1.9	0.5	5	0
(green beans (string beans), canned)	17	4.0	0.9	0.1	5	0

( ) indicates possible substitute foods that are lower in calories and/or fat.

Serving size--4 ounces:	Calories kcal	Carbo grams	Prot grams	Fat grams	Fat % of kcal	Chol mg
Corn, fresh	98	21.5	3.6	1.4	13	0
(green beans (string beans), fresh)	35	8.1	2.0	0.1	3	0
Corn pudding	124	14.5	5.0	6.0	44	104
(corn salad)	24	4.1	2.3	0.5	19	0
Corn salad	24	4.1	2.3	0.5	19	0
(iceberg lettuce)	15	2.4	1.1	0.2	12	0
Cowpeas, fresh	102	21.4	3.3	0.3	3	0
(green beans (string beans), fresh)	35	8.1	2.0	0.1	3	0
Cowpeas, leaf	33	5.4	4.6	0.3	8	0
(spinach, fresh)	25	4.0	3.3	0.3	11	0
Cucumber	15	3.3	0.6	0.1	6	0
(no alternate identified)						
Dandelion greens	51	10.4	3.1	0.8	14	0
(spinach, fresh)	25	4.0	3.3	0.3	11	0
Deviled eggs	286	1.6	11.5	25.6	81	521
(potato salad)	162	12.7	3.1	9.3	52	77
Dishcloth gourd	23	5.0	1.4	0.2	8	0
(white-flower gourd)	16	3.9	0.7	0	0	0
Dock, fresh	25	3.6	2.3	0.8	29	0
(watercress)	12	1.5	2.6	0.1	7	0
Dry lima beans, raw	391	72.6	23.1	1.8	4	0
(navy beans, canned)	76	14.7	6.9	0.8	9	0
Dry mung beans, raw	386	68.4	27.4	1.5	3	0
(navy beans, canned)	76	14.7	6.9	0.8	9	0
Dry pinto beans, raw	396	72.2	26.0	1.4	3	0
(navy beans, canned)	76	14.7	6.9	0.8	9	0
Egg salad	369	1.8	10.0	35.7	87	455
(potato salad)	162	12.7	3.1	9.3	52	77
Eggplant	29	7.1	1.2	0.1	3	0
(squash, zucchini)	16	3.3	1.4	0.1	6	0
Endive	19	3.7	1.5	0.2	9	0
(iceberg lettuce)	15	2.4	1.1	0.2	12	0
Eppaw	170	35.9	5.2	2.0	11	0
(green beans (string beans), fresh)	35	8.1	2.0	0.1	3	0

( ) indicates possible substitute foods that are lower in calories and/or fat.

Serving size--4 ounces:	Calories kcal	Carbo grams	Prot grams	Fat grams	Fat % of kcal	Chol mg
French fried potatoes/french fries	357	44.9	4.5	18.8	47	0
(potatoes, baked, without skin)	105	24.5	2.3	0.1	1	0
Fried potatoes/cottage fries	247	38.6	3.9	9.3	34	0
(potatoes, baked, without skin)	105	24.5	2.3	0.1	1	0
Fruit salad	57	14.7	0.6	0	0	0
(apricots, canned w/water wo/skin)	25	6.2	0.8	0	0	0
Garden cress	36	6.2	2.9	0.8	20	0
(watercress)	12	1.5	2.6	0.1	7	0
Garden salad (without dressing)	17	3.2	1.1	0.2	11	0
(no alternate identified)						
Garlic	169	37.5	7.3	0.6	3	0
(onions, fresh)	43	9.7	1.4	0.3	6	0
Ginger root	78	17.1	1.9	0.8	9	0
(coriander)	23	2.9	2.7	0.7	27	0
Green beans (string beans), canned	17	4.0	0.9	0.1	5	0
(no alternate identified)						
Green beans (string beans), fresh	35	8.1	2.0	0.1	3	0
(asparagus, fresh)	25	4.2	3.5	0.2	7	0
Green olives	132	1.5	1.6	14.4	98	0
(onions, fresh)	43	9.7	1.4	0.3	6	0
Green peas, canned	56	10.2	3.4	0.3	5	0
(green beans (string beans), canned)	17	4.0	0.9	0.1	5	0
Green peas, fresh	92	16.4	6.1	0.5	5	0
(green beans (string beans), fresh)	35	8.1	2.0	0.1	3	0
Green peppers (bell peppers)	31	7.3	1.0	0.2	5	0
(cucumber)	15	3.3	0.6	0.1	6	0
Ham salad	476	0.9	20.2	43.4	82	94
(ham, canned, extra-lean)	154	0.6	24	5.6	34	34
Hashed brown potatoes	238	25.4	3.1	14.5	53	15
(potatoes, baked, without skin)	105	24.5	2.3	0.1	1	0
Horseradish, raw	73	9.4	10.7	1.6	15	0
(hot chili peppers, raw)	45	10.8	2.3	0.2	4	0
Hot chili peppers, canned	28	6.9	1.0	0.1	3	0
(sweet pepper, canned)	20	4.4	0.9	0.3	13	0

( ) indicates possible substitute foods that are lower in calories and/or fat.

Serving size--4 ounces:	Calories kcal	Carbo grams	Prot grams	Fat grams	Fat % of kcal	Chol mg
Hot chili peppers, raw	45	10.8	2.3	0.2	4	0
(green peppers (bell peppers))	31	7.3	1.0	0.2	5	0
Hyacinth bean, seed, raw	383	69.2	25.2	1.7	4	0
(hyacinth beans)	52	10.4	2.4	0.2	3	0
Hyacinth beans	52	10.4	2.4	0.2	3	0
(green beans (string beans), fresh)	35	8.1	2.0	0.1	3	0
Iceberg lettuce	15	2.4	1.1	0.2	12	0
(watercress)	12	1.5	2.6	0.1	7	0
Instant mashed potatoes, cooked	128	17.0	2.2	6.4	45	16
(potatoes, baked, without skin)	105	24.5	2.3	0.1	1	0
Jalapeno peppers, canned	27	5.6	0.9	0.7	23	0
(no alternate identified)						
Jerusalem artichokes	86	19.7	2.3	0	0	0
(artichokes, fresh)	53	11.9	3.7	0.1	1	0
Kale, fresh	57	11.3	3.7	0.8	13	0
(spinach, fresh)	25	4.0	3.3	0.3	11	0
Kanpyo	293	73.7	9.8	0.7	2	0
(no alternate identified)						
Kidney beans, canned	96	17.7	6.0	0.3	3	0
(navy beans, canned)	76	14.7	6.9	0.8	9	0
Leeks	69	16.0	1.7	0.3	4	0
(onions, fresh)	43	9.7	1.4	0.3	6	0
Lentils	120	25.1	10.2	0.6	4	0
(green beans (string beans), fresh)	35	8.1	2.0	0.1	3	0
Lentils, whole, cooked	131	22.8	10.2	0.5	3	0
(green beans (string beans), fresh)	35	8.1	2.0	0.1	3	0
Lentils, whole, raw	383	64.7	31.8	1.1	3	0
(green beans (string beans), fresh)	35	8.1	2.0	0.1	3	0
Lima beans, canned	85	15.8	5.1	0.3	3	0
(green beans (string beans), canned)	17	4.0	0.9	0.1	5	0
Lima beans, fresh	128	22.9	7.7	1.0	7	0
(green beans (string beans), fresh)	35	8.1	2.0	0.1	3	0
Lobster salad	125	2.6	11.5	7.3	53	52
(shrimp cocktail)	108	17.8	8.5	0.6	5	59

( ) indicates possible substitute foods that are lower in calories and/or fat.

Serving size--4 ounces:	Calories kcal	Carbo grams	Prot grams	Fat grams	Fat % of kcal	Chol mg
Looseleaf lettuce	20	4.0	1.5	0.3	13	0
(iceberg lettuce)	15	2.4	1.1	0.2	12	0
Lotus root	64	19.5	2.9	0.1	1	0
(turnips, fresh)	31	7.0	1.0	0.1	3	0
Macaroni salad/pasta salad	331	19.2	3.1	27.3	74	20
(mixed vegetables, canned)	41	8.1	1.6	0.3	7	0
Mashed potatoes, w/milk & marg	120	18.9	2.2	4.8	36	2
(potatoes, baked, without skin)	105	24.5	2.3	0.1	1	0
Mixed vegetables, canned	41	8.1	1.6	0.3	7	0
(green beans (string beans), canned)	17	4.0	0.9	0.1	5	0
Mixed vegetables, frozen	73	15.3	3.7	0.6	7	0
(green beans (string beans), canned)	17	4.0	0.9	0.1	5	0
Mountain yams	76	18.5	1.5	0.1	1	0
(green beans (string beans), canned)	17	4.0	0.9	0.1	5	0
Mung bean sprouts, fresh	34	6.7	3.4	0.2	5	0
(taro shoots)	12	2.6	1.0	0.1	7	0
Mushrooms	28	5.2	2.4	0.5	16	0
(cucumber)	15	3.3	0.6	0.1	6	0
Mushrooms, canned	27	5.7	2.2	0.3	10	0
(cucumber)	15	3.3	0.6	0.1	6	0
Mushrooms, shiitake, cooked	62	16.2	1.8	0.2	4	0
(sweet pepper, canned)	20	4.4	0.9	0.3	13	0
Mustard greens	29	5.6	3.1	0.2	6	0
(watercress)	12	1.5	2.6	0.1	7	0
Mustard spinach	25	4.4	2.5	0.3	11	0
(new zealand spinach)	16	2.8	1.7	0.2	11	0
Navy beans, canned	76	14.7	6.9	0.8	9	0
(shellie beans, canned)	34	7.0	2.0	0.2	5	0
New zealand spinach	16	2.8	1.7	0.2	11	0
(watercress)	12	1.5	2.6	0.1	7	0
Okra	43	8.6	2.3	0.1	2	0
(new zealand spinach)	16	2.8	1.7	0.2	11	0
Olives (manzanilla)	146	2.9	1.2	15.6	96	0
(ripe olives (sevillan))	105	3.1	1.2	10.8	93	0

( ) indicates possible substitute foods that are lower in calories and/or fat.

Serving size--4 ounces:	Calories kcal	Carbo grams	Prot grams	Fat grams	Fat % of kcal	Chol mg
Onion rings	293	34.6	3.5	16.0	49	0
(potatoes, baked, without skin)	105	24.5	2.3	0.1	1	0
Onions, fresh	43	9.7	1.4	0.3	6	0
(spring onions)	36	8.3	2.0	0.2	4	0
Oriental radishes, dried	307	71.9	9.0	0.8	2	0
(oriental radishes, fresh)	20	4.6	0.7	0.1	4	0
Oriental radishes, fresh	20	4.6	0.7	0.1	4	0
(white icicle radish, fresh)	16	2.9	1.2	0.1	6	0
Pak-choi cabbage, fresh	15	2.5	1.7	0.2	12	0
(watercress)	12	1.5	2.6	0.1	7	0
Parsnips	85	20.4	1.4	0.3	3	0
(turnips, fresh)	31	7.0	1.0	0.1	3	0
Pe-tsai cabbage, fresh	18	3.6	1.4	0.2	10	0
(pak-choi cabbage, fresh)	15	2.5	1.7	0.2	12	0
Pea pods	48	8.6	3.2	0.2	4	0
(green beans (string beans), canned)	17	4.0	0.9	0.1	5	0
Peas and carrots, canned	43	9.6	2.5	0.3	6	0
(carrots, canned)	26	5.8	0.7	0.2	7	0
Peas and carrots, frozen	60	12.6	3.9	0.6	9	0
(carrots, canned)	26	5.8	0.7	0.2	7	0
Peas and onions, canned	58	9.8	3.7	0.5	8	0
(peas and carrots, canned)	43	9.6	2.5	0.3	6	0
Peas and onions, frozen	79	15.3	4.5	0.3	3	0
(peas and carrots, canned)	43	9.6	2.5	0.3	6	0
Peppers, sweet, stuffed	193	19.1	14.7	6.2	29	43
(sweet pepper, canned)	20	4.4	0.9	0.3	13	0
Pickle, chow-chow, sour	33	4.6	1.6	1.5	41	0
(pickle relish, sour)	22	3.1	0.8	1.0	41	0
Pickle, chow-chow, sweet	132	30.6	1.7	1.0	7	0
(pickle, chow-chow, sour)	33	4.6	1.6	1.5	41	0
Pickle, cucumber, dill	20	4.6	0.7	0.2	8	0
(pickle, cucumber, sour)	11	2.3	0.6	0.2	16	0
Pickle, cucumber, fresh	83	20.3	1.0	0.2	2	0
(pickle, cucumber, sour)	11	2.3	0.6	0.2	16	0

( ) indicates possible substitute foods that are lower in calories and/or fat.

Serving size--4 ounces:	Calories kcal	Carbo grams	Prot grams	Fat grams	Fat % of kcal	Chol mg
Pickle, cucumber, sour	11	2.3	0.6	0.2	16	0
(no alternate identified)						
Pickle, cucumber, sweet	133	36.0	0.5	0.3	2	0
(pickle, cucumber, sour)	11	2.3	0.6	0.2	16	0
Pickle relish, sour	22	3.1	0.8	1.0	41	0
(pickle, cucumber, sour)	11	2.3	0.6	0.2	16	0
Pickle relish, sweet	147	39.7	0.5	0.6	3	0
(pickle relish, sour)	22	3.1	0.8	1.0	41	0
Pickled beets, canned	74	18.5	0.9	0.1	1	0
(pickle, cucumber, sour)	11	2.3	0.6	0.2	16	0
Pigeonpeas	154	27.1	8.2	1.8	11	0
(green beans (string beans), canned)	17	4.0	0.9	0.1	5	0
Pimentos, canned	26	5.8	1.2	0.3	9	0
(sweet pepper, canned)	20	4.4	0.9	0.3	13	0
Pinto beans, canned	88	16.5	5.2	0.3	3	0
(navy beans, canned)	76	14.7	6.9	0.8	9	0
Poi	127	30.8	0.5	0.1	1	0
(taro, tahitian)	45	7.8	3.2	1.1	22	0
Pokeberry shoots	26	4.2	2.9	0.5	17	0
(taro shoots)	12	2.6	1.0	0.1	7	0
Potato chips	602	58.4	9.2	38.4	56	0
(pretzels)	432	89.7	10.3	4.0	8	0
Potato pancakes	308	32.4	7.0	17.2	50	109
(potatoes, baked, without skin)	105	24.5	2.3	0.1	1	0
Potato puffs	252	34.6	3.7	12.1	43	0
(potatoes, baked, without skin)	105	24.5	2.3	0.1	1	0
Potato salad	162	12.7	3.1	9.3	52	77
(potatoes, baked, without skin)	105	24.5	2.3	0.1	1	0
Potato skins, baked	225	52.3	4.9	0.1	0	0
(potatoes, baked, with skin)	124	28.6	2.6	0.1	1	0
Potato skins, deluxe, baked	295	30.6	12.6	13.8	42	34
(potatoes, baked, with skin)	124	28.6	2.6	0.1	1	0
Potato skins with cheese & bacon	336	33.0	14.3	16.4	44	41
(potatoes, baked, with skin)	124	28.6	2.6	0.1	1	0

( ) indicates possible substitute foods that are lower in calories and/or fat.

Serving size--4 ounces:	Calories kcal	Carbo grams	Prot grams	Fat grams	Fat % of kcal	Chol mg
Potato skins with cheese, baked	288	37.4	11.5	10.7	33	34
(potatoes, baked, with skin)	124	28.6	2.6	0.1	1	0
Potato sticks	592	60.4	7.6	39.1	59	0
(pretzels)	432	89.7	10.3	4.0	8	0
Potatoes, au gratin	150	12.8	5.8	8.6	52	26
(scalloped potatoes)	98	12.2	3.3	4.2	39	14
Potatoes, baked, with skin	124	28.6	2.6	0.1	1	0
(potatoes, baked, without skin)	105	24.5	2.3	0.1	1	0
Potatoes, baked, without skin	105	24.5	2.3	0.1	1	0
(green beans (string beans), fresh)	35	8.1	2.0	0.1	3	0
Potatoes, boiled	99	22.8	2.2	0.1	1	0
(green beans (string beans), canned)	17	4.0	0.9	0.1	5	0
Potatoes, canned	45	9.9	1.6	0.1	2	0
(green beans (string beans), canned)	17	4.0	0.9	0.1	5	0
Poultry salad spread	227	8.4	13.2	15.3	61	34
(turkey loaf breast)	125	0	25.5	1.8	13	46
Pumpkin, canned	39	9.2	1.2	0.3	7	0
(pumpkin, raw)	29	7.4	1.1	0.1	3	0
Pumpkin flowers	17	3.7	1.1	0.1	5	0
(watercress)	12	1.5	2.6	0.1	7	0
Pumpkin leaves	22	2.6	3.5	0.5	20	0
(purslane)	18	3.9	1.5	0.1	5	0
Pumpkin pie mix, canned	118	29.9	1.2	0.1	1	0
(pumpkin, canned)	39	9.2	1.2	0.3	7	0
Pumpkin, raw	29	7.4	1.1	0.1	3	0
(squash, summer)	23	4.9	1.4	0.2	8	0
Purslane	18	3.9	1.5	0.1	5	0
(watercress)	12	1.5	2.6	0.1	7	0
Radish sprouts	49	4.1	4.3	2.8	51	0
(mung bean sprouts, fresh)	34	6.7	3.4	0.2	5	0
Radishes, fresh	19	4.1	0.7	0.6	28	0
(white icicle radish, fresh)	16	2.9	1.2	0.1	6	0
Red cabbage, fresh	31	6.9	1.6	0.3	9	0
(pak-choi cabbage, fresh)	15	2.5	1.7	0.2	12	0

( ) indicates possible substitute foods that are lower in calories and/or fat.

Serving size--4 ounces:	Calories kcal	Carbo grams	Prot grams	Fat grams	Fat % of kcal	Chol mg
Refried beans	121	21.0	7.0	1.2	9	0
(navy beans, canned)	76	14.7	6.9	0.8	9	0
Rhubarb	24	5.1	1.0	0.2	7	0
(watercress)	12	1.5	2.6	0.1	7	0
Ripe olives (ascolano)	146	2.9	1.2	15.6	96	0
(ripe olives (sevillan))	105	3.1	1.2	10.8	93	0
Ripe olives (mission)	209	3.6	1.4	22.8	98	0
(ripe olives (sevillan))	105	3.1	1.2	10.8	93	0
Ripe olives (sevillan)	105	3.1	1.2	10.8	93	0
(pickle, cucumber, dill)	20	4.6	0.7	0.2	8	0
Ripe olives, salt cured	383	9.9	2.5	40.6	95	0
(ripe olives (sevillan))	105	3.1	1.2	10.8	93	0
Romain lettuce	18	2.7	1.8	0.2	10	0
(iceberg lettuce)	15	2.4	1.1	0.2	12	0
Rutabagas	41	9.2	1.4	0.2	4	0
(turnips, fresh)	31	7.0	1.0	0.1	3	0
Salad with egg and cheese	53	2.5	4.5	3.1	53	46
(tossed salad (without dressing))	17	3.2	1.1	0.2	11	0
Salad w/turkey, ham and cheese	93	1.6	9.1	5.6	54	49
(tossed salad (without dressing))	17	3.2	1.1	0.2	11	0
Salsify	93	21.1	3.7	0.2	2	0
(beets, fresh)	50	11.3	1.7	0.1	2	0
Sauerkraut	22	4.9	1.0	0.1	4	0
(pickle, cucumber, sour)	11	2.3	0.6	0.2	16	0
Savoy cabbage, fresh	31	6.9	2.3	0.1	3	0
(pak-choi cabbage, fresh)	15	2.5	1.7	0.2	12	0
Scalloped potatoes	98	12.2	3.3	4.2	39	14
(green beans (string beans), canned)	17	4.0	0.9	0.1	5	0
Scotch kale, fresh	48	9.4	3.2	0.7	13	0
(spinach, fresh)	25	4.0	3.3	0.3	11	0
Seafood salad	201	2.0	12.1	16.0	72	67
(shrimp cocktail)	108	17.8	8.5	0.6	5	59
Seaweed, agar, dried	347	91.7	7.0	0.3	1	0
(seaweed, agar, fresh)	29	7.7	0.6	0	0	0

( ) indicates possible substitute foods that are lower in calories and/or fat.

Serving size--4 ounces:	Calories kcal	Carbo grams	Prot grams	Fat grams	Fat % of kcal	Chol mg
Seaweed, agar, fresh	29	7.7	0.6	0	0	0
(watercress)	12	1.5	2.6	0.1	7	0
Seaweed, irish moss, fresh	56	13.9	1.7	0.2	3	0
(seaweed, agar, fresh)	29	7.7	0.6	0	0	0
Seaweed, kelp, fresh	49	10.9	1.9	0.7	13	0
(seaweed, agar, fresh)	29	7.7	0.6	0	0	0
Seaweed, laver, fresh	40	5.8	6.6	0.3	7	0
(seaweed, agar, fresh)	29	7.7	0.6	0	0	0
Seaweed, spirulina, dried	329	27.1	65.2	8.7	24	0
(seaweed, spirulina, fresh)	29	2.7	6.7	0.5	16	0
Seaweed, spirulina, fresh	29	2.7	6.7	0.5	16	0
(watercress)	12	1.5	2.6	0.1	7	0
Seaweed, wakame, fresh	51	10.3	3.4	0.7	12	0
(seaweed, agar, fresh)	29	7.7	0.6	0	0	0
Sesbania flower	31	7.6	1.5	0	0	0
(pumpkin flowers)	17	3.7	1.1	0.1	5	0
Shallots, raw	82	19.1	2.8	0.1	1	0
(onions, fresh)	43	9.7	1.4	0.3	6	0
Shellie beans, canned	34	7.0	2.0	0.2	5	0
(green beans (string beans), canned)	17	4.0	0.9	0.1	5	0
Shrimp salad	179	2.6	12.0	13.3	67	106
(shrimp cocktail)	108	17.8	8.5	0.6	5	59
Soybeans	167	12.5	14.6	7.7	41	0
(navy beans, canned)	76	14.7	6.9	0.8	9	0
Spinach, canned	22	3.3	2.4	0.5	20	0
(watercress)	12	1.5	2.6	0.1	7	0
Spinach, fresh	25	4.0	3.3	0.3	11	0
(endive)	19	3.7	1.5	0.2	9	0
Spinach salad (without dressing)	25	4.4	2.8	0.2	7	0
(tossed salad (without dressing))	17	3.2	1.1	0.2	11	0
Spring onions	36	8.3	2.0	0.2	4	0
(no alternate identified)						
Sprouted peas	145	32.1	10.0	0.8	5	0
(green beans (string beans), fresh)	35	8.1	2.0	0.1	3	0

( ) indicates possible substitute foods that are lower in calories and/or fat.

Serving size--4 ounces:	Calories kcal	Carbo grams	Prot grams	Fat grams	Fat % of kcal	Chol mg
Squash, acorn	45	11.8	0.9	0.1	2	0
(squash, summer)	23	4.9	1.4	0.2	8	0
Squash, butternut	51	13.3	1.1	0.1	2	0
(squash, crookneck)	22	4.5	1.0	0.2	8	0
Squash, crookneck	22	4.5	1.0	0.2	8	0
(squash, zucchini)	16	3.3	1.4	0.1	6	0
Squash, hubbard	45	9.9	2.3	0.6	12	0
(squash, scallop)	20	4.3	1.4	0.2	9	0
Squash, scallop	20	4.3	1.4	0.2	9	0
(squash, zucchini)	16	3.3	1.4	0.1	6	0
Squash, spaghetti	37	7.8	0.7	0.7	17	0
(squash, summer)	23	4.9	1.4	0.2	8	0
Squash, summer	23	4.9	1.4	0.2	8	0
(squash, zucchini)	16	3.3	1.4	0.1	6	0
Squash, winter	42	10.0	1.6	0.2	4	0
(squash, summer)	23	4.9	1.4	0.2	8	0
Squash, zucchini	16	3.3	1.4	0.1	6	0
(cucumber)	15	3.3	0.6	0.1	6	0
Stewed tomatoes, canned	29	7.4	1.0	0.1	3	0
(sweet pepper, canned)	20	4.4	0.9	0.3	13	0
Succotash, canned	71	15.9	2.9	0.6	8	0
(squash, zucchini)	16	3.3	1.4	0.1	6	0
Succotash, fresh	112	22.2	5.7	1.1	9	0
(squash, zucchini)	16	3.3	1.4	0.1	6	0
Swamp cabbage	22	3.5	2.9	0.2	8	0
(watercress)	12	1.5	2.6	0.1	7	0
Sweet pepper, canned	20	4.4	0.9	0.3	13	0
(cucumber)	15	3.3	0.6	0.1	6	0
Sweet pepper, fresh	31	7.3	1.0	0.2	5	0
(cucumber)	15	3.3	0.6	0.1	6	0
Sweet potato leaves	40	7.3	4.5	0.3	7	0
(spinach, fresh)	25	4.0	3.3	0.3	11	0
Sweet potatoes, candied	155	31.6	1.0	3.7	21	9
(sweet potatoes, fresh)	119	27.6	1.8	0.3	2	0

( ) indicates possible substitute foods that are lower in calories and/or fat.

Serving size--4 ounces:	Calories kcal	Carbo grams	Prot grams	Fat grams	Fat % of kcal	Chol mg
Sweet potatoes, canned	103	23.9	1.8	0.2	2	0
(mountain yams)	76	18.5	1.5	0.1	1	0
Sweet potatoes, fresh	119	27.6	1.8	0.3	2	0
(mountain yams)	76	18.5	1.5	0.1	1	0
Swiss chard	22	4.2	2.0	0.2	8	0
(watercress)	12	1.5	2.6	0.1	7	0
Taro chips	564	77.2	2.6	28.2	44	0
(taro, fresh)	121	30.1	1.7	0.2	1	0
Taro, fresh	121	30.1	1.7	0.2	1	0
(taro shoots)	12	2.6	1.0	0.1	7	0
Taro leaves	48	7.6	5.7	0.8	15	0
(taro shoots)	12	2.6	1.0	0.1	7	0
Taro shoots	12	2.6	1.0	0.1	7	0
(no alternate identified)						
Taro, tahitian	45	7.8	3.2	1.1	22	0
(taro shoots)	12	2.6	1.0	0.1	7	0
Tofu	86	2.2	9.2	5.4	56	0
(bamboo shoots, fresh)	31	5.9	2.9	0.3	9	0
Tomato juice	19	4.8	0.9	0.1	5	0
(no alternate identified)						
Tomato paste, canned	95	21.3	4.3	1.0	9	0
(tomato sauce, canned)	34	8.2	1.5	0.2	5	0
Tomato puree, canned	46	11.3	1.9	0.1	2	0
(tomato sauce, canned)	34	8.2	1.5	0.2	5	0
Tomato sauce, canned	34	8.2	1.5	0.2	5	0
(tomatoes, whole, canned)	23	4.9	1.0	0.2	8	0
Tomatoes, red, ripe	22	4.9	1.0	0.2	8	0
(cucumber)	15	3.3	0.6	0.1	6	0
Tomatoes, whole, canned	23	4.9	1.0	0.2	8	0
(cucumber)	15	3.3	0.6	0.1	6	0
Tossed salad (without dressing)	17	3.2	1.1	0.2	11	0
(watercress)	12	1.5	2.6	0.1	7	0
Tree fern	45	12.5	0.3	0.1	2	0
(turnip greens, fresh)	31	6.5	1.7	0.3	9	0

( ) indicates possible substitute foods that are lower in calories and/or fat.

Serving size--4 ounces:	Calories kcal	Carbo grams	Prot grams	Fat grams	Fat % of kcal	Chol mg
Tuna salad	193	4.0	16.6	11.9	55	74
(tuna fish, canned in water)	144	0	31.8	0.9	6	71
Turnip greens, canned	16	2.7	1.6	0.3	17	0
(watercress)	12	1.5	2.6	0.1	7	0
Turnip greens, fresh	31	6.5	1.7	0.3	9	0
(spinach, fresh)	25	4.0	3.3	0.3	11	0
Turnips, fresh	31	7.0	1.0	0.1	3	0
(squash, zucchini)	16	3.3	1.4	0.1	6	0
Vegetable juice cocktail	22	5.1	0.7	0.1	4	0
(tomato juice)	19	4.8	0.9	0.1	5	0
Vine spinach	22	3.9	2.0	0.3	12	0
(watercress)	12	1.5	2.6	0.1	7	0
Water chestnuts, canned	57	14.1	1.0	0.1	2	0
(bamboo shoots, canned)	22	3.6	1.9	0.5	20	0
Water chestnuts, fresh	120	27.1	1.6	0.1	1	0
(bamboo shoots, fresh)	31	5.9	2.9	0.3	9	0
Watercress	12	1.5	2.6	0.1	7	0
(no alternate identified)						
Waxgourd	15	3.4	0.5	0.2	12	0
(no alternate identified)						
Welsh onions	39	7.4	2.2	0.5	12	0
(spring onions)	36	8.3	2.0	0.2	4	0
White-flower gourd	16	3.9	0.7	0	0	0
(no alternate identified)						
White icicle radish, fresh	16	2.9	1.2	0.1	6	0
(cucumber)	15	3.3	0.6	0.1	6	0
Winged bean leaves	84	16.0	6.6	1.2	13	0
(winged beans)	56	4.9	7.8	1.0	16	0
Winged beans	56	4.9	7.8	1.0	16	0
(green beans (string beans), canned)	17	4.0	0.9	0.1	5	0
Witloof chicory	17	3.6	1.1	0.1	5	0
(watercress)	12	1.5	2.6	0.1	7	0
Yambeans	46	10.0	1.6	0.2	4	0
(green beans (string beans), canned)	17	4.0	0.9	0.1	5	0

( ) indicates possible substitute foods that are lower in calories and/or fat.

Serving size--4 ounces:	Calories kcal	Carbo grams	Prot grams	Fat grams	Fat % of kcal	Chol mg
Yams, fresh	134	31.6	1.7	0.2	1	0
(mountain yams)	76	18.5	1.5	0.1	1	0
Yardlong beans	53	9.4	3.2	0.5	8	0
(green beans (string beans), canned)	17	4.0	0.9	0.1	5	0

( ) indicates possible substitute foods that are lower in calories and/or fat.

NUTRITION TABLES

This chapter is a tool for finding good sources of certain vitamins and minerals. For example, while TV ads may lead us to believe oranges, milk and bananas are the best sources for vitamin C, calcium and potassium, respectively, our tables show otherwise.

Our tables of nutritional data are derived from two sources. The information on RDA's, adequate and safe levels of consumption, and attributes of vitamins, minerals and trace elements comes from *Recommended Dietary Allowances*, tenth edition, by the Food and Nutrition Board of the National Research Council. The vitamin, mineral and other nutritional content of certain foods is derived from the *USDA Nutrient Data Base for Standard Reference*. See the Selected Bibliography.

Please note that our tables do not include all vitamins, minerals and trace elements, and the foods presented in the tables represent a selected listing rather than a comprehensive listing. All foods in our tables are fresh/raw unless otherwise specified.

The foods we have included in our nutrition tables are naturally high in the nutrients indicated. There are other foods that are fortified or enriched that could serve as good sources for vitamins and minerals. In particular, certain breakfast cereals contain 100% of the Recommended Dietary Allowance for many different vitamins and minerals. The nutritional content of breakfast cereals and other fortified or enriched products is printed on their packaging. Also, our nutrition tables do not include a variety of herbs, spices and dehydrated foods because their normal serving sizes are a small fraction of the 3.5-ounce serving size used in the tables.

The information presented in our tables is intended for adults with no special dietary needs or restrictions. If you are pregnant, lactating, younger than 19, or otherwise have special needs, it is important that you obtain additional guidance from your doctor or dietitian. Also, it is important to note that large quantities of many vitamins and minerals are toxic. Therefore, logically, if you are consuming foods high in those vitamins and minerals, it is unlikely that supplements are appropriate. Consult your physician.

VITAMIN C (ascorbic acid)

Vitamin C is an antioxidant that may affect immune responses and wound healing and plays a role in numerous biochemical processes in the human body. A prolonged deficiency in vitamin C will eventually lead to scurvy, a serious disease characterized by widespread capillary hemorrhaging. The Food and Nutrition Board of the National Research Council has determined that the Recommended Dietary Allowance of vitamin C for adults is 60 mg per day. The Food and Nutrition Board also recommends that regular cigarette smokers consume a minimum of 100 mg per day. Heat and water used in cooking cause a significant loss of vitamin C from foods.

Food Description	mg per 3.5 ounces	% of RDA
Acerola	1678	2797%
Acerola juice	1600	2667%
Hot chili pepper	243	405%
Sweet red peppers	190	317%
Guavas, common	184	307%
Kale	130	217%
Mustard spinach	130	217%
Kiwifruit	98	163%
Taro, Tahitian	96	160%
Broccoli	93	155%
Parsley	90	150%
Brussels sprouts	85	142%
Chives	79	132%
Cauliflower	72	120%
Papayas	62	103%
Strawberries	57	95%
Orange	53	88%
Lemon	53	88%
Orange juice	50	83%
Grapefruit	38	63%
Lime	29	48%
Spinach	28	47%

VITAMIN A

Vitamin A (retinol and carotenoids) is essential for vision, growth, reproduction and immune system functions. Vitamin A deficiency can cause night blindness and severe eye disorders. The Food and Nutrition Board of the National Research Council has determined that the Recommended Dietary Allowance of vitamin A for adult males is 1000 RE (3333 IU) and for adult females is 800 RE (2667 IU) per day.

WARNING: Extremely high doses of vitamin A (retinol) are toxic.

Units of measurement and conversion:
1 RE = 1 μg of all-trans retinol = 6 μg all-trans ß-carotene = 3 1/3 IU.

Food Description	IU per 3.5 ounces	% RDA for adult: males	females
Duck liver	39907	1197%	1497%
Beef liver	35346	1060%	1325%
Carrots	28129	844%	1055%
Carrot juice, canned	25751	773%	966%
Pumpkin, canned	22056	662%	827%
Chicken liver	20549	616%	771%
Sweet potato	20063	602%	752%
Broccoli leaves	16000	480%	600%
Dandelion greens	14000	420%	525%
Shallots	12484	375%	468%
Hot chili pepper	10750	323%	403%
Mustard spinach	9900	297%	371%
Garden cress	9300	279%	349%
Kale	8900	267%	334%
Spinach, canned, drained	8776	263%	329%
Cantaloupe	3224	97%	121%
Apricots	2612	78%	98%
Tomatoes, red, ripe	623	19%	23%

CALCIUM

Calcium is essential for the development and maintenance of strong bones. Lack of calcium in the diet, especially during childhood through age 25, is associated with bone loss and osteoporosis later in life. Vitamin D aids in the absorption of calcium. The Food and Nutrition Board of the National Research Council has determined that the Recommended Dietary Allowance of calcium is 1200 mg per day for male and female adolescents through age 24 years. For adults age 25 and older, the Board's RDA is 800 mg per day.

Food Description	mg per 3.5 ounces	% of RDA by age: 11 - 24	25+ yrs.
Hard parmesan cheese	1184	99%	148%
Romano cheese	1064	89%	133%
Swiss cheese	961	80%	120%
Provolone cheese	756	63%	95%
Cheddar cheese	721	60%	90%
Blue cheese	528	44%	66%
Feta cheese	493	41%	62%
Tahini kernels	420	35%	53%
Sardines canned w/oil, drained	382	32%	48%
Crab, baked	381	32%	48%
Crab cake	337	28%	42%
Seaweed, dulce	296	25%	37%
Almonds, dry roasted	282	24%	35%
Soybeans	277	23%	35%
Caviar	275	23%	34%
Cheese pizza	221	18%	28%
Mustard spinach	210	18%	26%
Turnip greens	190	16%	24%
Brie cheese	184	15%	23%
Garlic	181	15%	23%
Anchovy	147	12%	18%
Skim milk	123	10%	15%
Whole milk	119	10%	15%

POTASSIUM

Potassium is an electrolyte that plays an essential role in nerve-pulse transmissions, skeletal muscle functioning and maintenance of normal blood pressure. Potassium is present in a wide range of foods, and potassium deficiency does not occur under normal circumstances. The Food and Nutrition Board of the National Research Council has not established a Recommended Dietary Allowance for potassium, but the Board states that the minimum requirement is approximately 1600 to 2000 mg per day.

WARNING: Extremely high doses of potassium are toxic.

Food Description	mg per 3.5 ounces	% of 2000
Soybeans	1797	90%
White beans	1795	90%
Shiitake mushroom, dried	1534	77%
Kidney beans	1406	70%
Pinto beans	1328	66%
Potato chips	1298	65%
Pistachio nut, dry roasted	970	49%
Pineapple, candied	944	47%
Lentils	905	45%
Chickpeas	875	44%
Yams	816	41%
Almonds, dry roasted	770	39%
Raisins, seedless	751	38%
Prunes, dried	745	37%
Fig, dried	712	36%
Rainbow trout, baked/broiled	634	32%
Clams	628	31%
Avocado	599	30%
Chestnuts, European, roasted	592	30%
Water chestnut, Chinese	584	29%
Spinach	558	28%
Bananas	396	20%

IRON

Iron is an essential trace element that is widely present in foods consumed in the United States. Severe iron deficiency causes decreased work capacity and anemia and has been associated with a decreased function of the immune system. The Food and Nutrition Board of the National Research Council has determined that the Recommended Dietary Allowance of iron for adult males is 10 mg per day and for adult females is 15 mg per day (except women over the age of 50 have an RDA of 10 mg per day).

WARNING: High doses of iron are toxic, especially for young children.

Food Description	mg per 3.5 ounces	% RDA for adult:	
		males	females
Beef spleen	45	450%	300%
Lamb spleen	42	420%	280%
Goose liver	31	310%	207%
Duck liver	31	310%	207%
Seaweed, spirulina, drained	29	290%	193%
Clams, boiled or steamed	28	280%	187%
Pork liver	23	230%	153%
Pork spleen	22	220%	147%
Pork lungs	19	190%	127%
Soybeans	16	160%	107%
Pumpkin kernel, roasted	15	150%	100%
Winged bean	13	130%	87%
Oysters, boiled or steamed	13	130%	87%
Caviar	12	120%	80%
Turkey liver	11	110%	73%
Tofu	10	100%	67%
White beans	10	100%	67%
Lentils	9	90%	60%
Seaweed, Irish moss	9	90%	60%

MANGANESE

Manganese is a trace element essential for normal growth, bone and cartilage formation, and reproduction processes (including fetal development). Because of its widespread presence in foods and the relatively low manganese requirement in our diets, manganese deficiency is rare. The Food and Nutrition Board of the National Research Council has determined that the estimated safe and adequate daily dietary intake of manganese for adults is 2 to 5 mg per day. No RDA has been established.

WARNING: High doses of manganese are toxic.

Food Description	mg per 3.5 ounces	% of 3 mg
Oysters, eastern	91	3033%
Oysters, pacific	17	567%
Beef shank, lean, simmered	10	333%
Tahini kernels	10	333%
Pumpkin seeds, roasted	10	333%
Beef blade, lean, braised	10	333%
Hyacinth beans	9	300%
Beef arm, lean, braised	9	300%
Lamb, lean, cooked	9	300%
Mushroom, shiitake, dried	8	267%
King crab, boiled/steamed	8	267%
Lamb liver, braised	8	267%
Chicken heart, simmered	7	233%
Turkey neck, w/o skin, simmered	7	233%
Beef tip round, roasted	7	233%
Beef sirloin, lean, broiled	7	233%
Peanuts, oil roasted	7	233%
Crab, baked	6	200%
Spiny lobster	6	200%
Pecans and cashews, dry roasted	6	200%
Almonds, dry roasted	5	167%

VITAMIN E (alpha-tocopherol)

Vitamin E is an antioxidant. It helps prevent potentially harmful oxidations that can damage cells. Although vitamin E deficiency does not normally occur, deficiency can cause reproductive failure and neurological abnormalities. The Food and Nutrition Board of the National Research Council has determined that the Recommended Dietary Allowance of vitamin E for adult males is 10 mg per day, and for adult females is 8 mg per day. Processing, storage and cooking cause some loss of vitamin E from foods.

Food Description	mg per 3.5 ounces (alpha-tocopherol)	% RDA for adult: males	females
Wheat germ oil	149	1490%	1863%
Sunflower oil	60	600%	750%
Hazelnut oil	47	470%	588%
Almond oil	39	390%	488%
Cottonseed oil	35	350%	438%
Safflower oil	34	340%	425%
Grape seed oil	29	290%	363%
Mayonnaise, safflower/soybean	22	220%	275%
Corn oil	14	140%	175%
Olive oil	12	120%	150%
Peanut oil	12	120%	150%
Hard margarine	9	90%	113%
Peanuts	8	80%	100%
Soft margarine	7	70%	88%
Blue cheese salad dressing	6	60%	75%
Russian salad dressing	6	60%	75%
French salad dressing	5	50%	63%
Italian salad dressing	5	50%	63%
Thousand island salad dressing	4	40%	50%
Navy beans	4	40%	50%
Chicken fat	3	30%	38%
Avocado	1	40%	50%
Mango	1	10%	13%

THIAMIN (vitamin B_1)

Thiamin deficiency over a prolonged period results in beriberi, a disease of the nervous and cardiovascular systems. The Food and Nutrition Board of the National Research Council has determined that the Recommended Dietary Allowance of thiamin for adults is 0.5 mg per 1000 kcal, with a minimum of 1.0 mg per day.

Food Description	mg per 3.5 ounces	% of 1 mg
Rice bran, crude	2.8	280%
Seaweed, spirulina	2.4	240%
Sunflower kernel, dried	2.3	230%
Tahini kernels	1.6	160%
Pork centerloin, lean	1.2	120%
Oat bran	1.2	120%
Hyacinth beans	1.1	110%
Pork sirloin, lean	1.1	110%
Winged beans	1.0	100%
Pork tenderloin	1.0	100%
Ham, cured, lean	0.9	90%
Dry salami, pork	0.9	90%
Black beans	0.9	90%
Yardlong beans	0.9	90%
Soybeans	0.9	90%
Cowpeas	0.9	90%
Canadian bacon, cooked	0.8	80%
Oats	0.8	80%
Split peas	0.7	70%
Smoked link sausage	0.7	70%
Bacon, cured, cooked	0.7	70%
Navy beans	0.6	60%
Peanuts	0.6	60%
Lamb kidneys	0.6	60%
Kidney beans, red	0.6	60%

RIBOFLAVIN (vitamin B_2)

Riboflavin is essential for niacin and vitamin B_6 to function properly in the human body. Riboflavin deficiency symptoms include skin disorders and a range of difficulties associated with deficiency of niacin and vitamin B_6. The Food and Nutrition Board of the National Research Council has determined that the Recommended Dietary Allowance of riboflavin for adults through age 50 is 1.7 mg for males and 1.3 mg for females. After age 50, the RDA's decrease to 1.4 mg and 1.2 mg for males and females respectively.

Food Description	mg per 3.5 ounces	% RDA (age<51) males	females
Lamb liver	3.6	212%	277%
Pork liver	3.0	177%	231%
Beef liver	2.8	165%	215%
Beef kidneys	2.6	153%	200%
Lamb kidneys	2.2	129%	169%
Turkey liver	2.2	129%	169%
Chicken liver	2.0	118%	154%
Pork kidneys	1.7	100%	131%
Braunschweiger, pork	1.5	88%	115%
Gjetost cheese	1.4	82%	108%
Pork heart	1.2	71%	92%
Almonds, oil roasted	1.0	59%	77%
Soybeans	0.9	53%	69%
Feta cheese	0.8	47%	62%
Caviar	0.6	35%	46%
Winged bean leaves	0.6	35%	46%
Liver pate	0.6	35%	46%
Scallops, breaded, fried	0.6	35%	46%
Roquefort cheese	0.6	35%	46%
Shrimp, breaded, fried	0.6	35%	46%
Eggs, chicken	0.5	29%	38%
Brie cheese	0.5	29%	38%
Mixed nuts	0.5	29%	38%

NIACIN (B-complex vitamin)

Niacin plays a role in various metabolic functions. A deficiency in niacin can lead to pellagra, a disease affecting the skin and digestive system. In severe cases, pellagra can cause mental deterioration and dementia. The Food and Nutrition Board of the National Research Council has determined that the Recommended Dietary Allowance of niacin for adults is 6.6 NEs per 1000 kcal, with a minimum of 13 NEs per day. (1 NE = 1 niacin equivalent = 1 mg niacin or 60 mg tryptophan). Cooking and storage do not significantly reduce the amount of niacin in foods.

WARNING: High doses of niacin may produce vascular dilation and may result in various metabolic effects.

Food Description	mg per 3.5 ounces	% of 13 mg
Anchovy, canned in oil, drained	20	154%
Lamb liver	16	123%
Spanish peanuts	16	123%
Pork liver	15	115%
Shiitake mushroom, dried	14	108%
Pacific barracuda	13	100%
Peanut butter	13	100%
Seaweed, spirulina, drained	13	100%
Beef liver	13	100%
Tuna, canned w/water, drained	12	92%
Smoked sturgeon	11	85%
Chicken, light meat	10	77%
Turkey liver	10	77%
Tuna, yellowfin	10	77%
Swordfish	10	77%
Beef heart	9	69%
Chicken liver	9	69%
Mackerel, Atlantic	9	69%
Veal, loin, lean	9	69%
Braunschweiger, pork	8	62%

PANTOTHENIC ACID (B-complex vitamin)

Pantothenic acid is a B-complex vitamin that aids in a variety of biochemical processes involving growth and reproduction. Because pantothenic acid is widely distributed in foods, deficiency does not normally occur. The Food and Nutrition Board of the National Research Council has determined that the estimated safe and adequate daily dietary intake of pantothenic acid for adults is 4 to 7 mg per day.

Food Description	mg per 3.5 ounces	% of 5 mg
Mushroom, shiitake, dried	21.9	438%
Turkey liver	7.7	154%
Beef liver	7.7	154%
Sunflower kernel, toasted	7.1	142%
Sunflower seed butter	7.0	140%
Pork liver	6.7	134%
Chicken liver	6.2	124%
Duck liver	6.2	124%
Goose liver	6.2	124%
Lamb liver	6.1	122%
Pork pancreas	4.6	92%
Lamb kidney	4.2	84%
Turkey giblets	4.0	80%
Beef pancreas	3.9	78%
Egg yolk, chicken	3.8	76%
Beef kidney	3.6	72%
Liver cheese, pork	3.5	70%
Caviar	3.5	70%
Seaweed, spirulina	3.5	70%
Braunschweiger, pork	3.4	68%
Chicken giblets	3.0	60%
Abalone	3.0	60%
Pork brains	2.8	56%
Turkey heart	2.7	54%
Chicken liver pate	2.6	52%

FOLATE

Folate aids in a variety of biochemical processes, including cell division and protein synthesis. Folate is widely present in foods, but cooking, processing and storing destroys as much as 50% of the folate present in foods. The Food and Nutrition Board of the National Research Council has determined that the Recommended Dietary Allowance of folate for adult males is 200 μg per day, and for adult females is 180 μg per day.

Food Description	μg per 3.5 ounces	% RDA for adult: males	females
Chicken liver	738	369%	410%
Turkey liver	738	369%	410%
Duck liver	738	369%	410%
Goose liver	738	369%	410%
Yardlong beans	658	329%	366%
Cowpeas	633	317%	352%
Mung beans	625	313%	347%
Chickpeas	557	279%	309%
Pinto beans	506	253%	281%
Black beans	444	222%	247%
Lentils	433	217%	241%
Broadbeans	423	212%	235%
Lima beans	398	199%	221%
Kidney beans	394	197%	219%
Soybeans	375	188%	208%
Navy beans	369	185%	205%
Chicken giblets	345	173%	192%
Split peas	274	137%	152%
Beef liver	248	124%	138%
Peanuts	240	120%	133%
Sunflower kernels, roasted	237	119%	132%
Turnip greens	194	97%	108%
Spinach	194	97%	108%

VITAMIN B_6

Vitamin B_6 aids in the metabolism of amino acids. A deficiency in vitamin B_6 can cause skin disorders, anemia and convulsions. Food processing, including freezing, results in considerable loss of the vitamin from the food. The Food and Nutrition Board of the National Research Council has determined that the Recommended Dietary Allowance of vitamin B_6 for adult males is 2 mg per day, and for adult females is 1.6 mg per day.

WARNING: Extremely high doses of vitamin B_6 (e.g., gram quantities for months or years) can be toxic.

Food Description	mg per 3.5 ounces	% RDA for adult: males	females
Garlic	1.2	60%	75%
Shiitake mushroom, dried	1.0	50%	63%
Beef liver	0.9	45%	56%
Lamb liver	0.9	45%	56%
Tuna, yellowfin	0.9	45%	56%
Salmon, Atlantic	0.8	40%	50%
Sunflower kernel, roasted	0.8	40%	50%
Turkey liver	0.8	40%	50%
Chicken liver	0.8	40%	50%
Duck liver	0.8	40%	50%
Goose liver	0.8	40%	50%
Pork liver	0.7	35%	44%
Pheasant	0.7	35%	44%
Taro chips	0.7	35%	44%
Goose meat	0.6	30%	38%
Filberts, dry roasted	0.6	30%	38%
Corn	0.6	30%	38%
Potatoes, baked with skin	0.6	30%	38%
Chicken breast, no skin	0.6	30%	38%
Bananas	0.6	30%	38%
Mayonnaise	0.6	30%	38%

VITAMIN B_{12}

Vitamin B_{12} plays a role in metabolic processes. Deficiency of vitamin B_{12} results in anemia and nervous system disorders. The Food and Nutrition Board of the National Research Council has determined that the Recommended Dietary Allowance of vitamin B_{12} for adults is 2.0 μg per day. Vitamin B_{12} is not destroyed by heat from cooking food.

Food Description	μg per 3.5 ounces	% of RDA
Lamb liver	90	4500%
Beef liver	69	3450%
Turkey liver	63	3150%
Goose or goose liver	54	2700%
Clams	49	2450%
Clam and tomato juice,canned	31	1550%
Beef kidneys	27	1350%
Pork liver	26	1300%
Chicken liver	23	1150%
Braunschweiger, pork	20	1000%
Octopus	20	1000%
Caviar	20	1000%
Oysters	19	950%
Mackerel, King	16	800%
Crab, baked	14	700%
Herring, Atlantic	14	700%
Mussels	12	600%
Chicken giblets	11	550%
Tuna, bluefin	9	450%
Sardines, canned, drained	9	450%
Dungeness or blue crab	9	450%
Alaska king crab	9	450%
Chicken liver pate	8	400%
Pork kidneys	8	400%
Trout	8	400%
Bluefish	5	250%

SELECTED BIBLIOGRAPHY

Adams, Catherine F. *Nutritive Value of American Foods in Common Units.* Agriculture Handbook 456. Agricultural Research Service. United States Department of Agriculture. Washington, DC: GPO, 1975.

Altman, Philip L. and Dorothy S. Dittmer, eds. *Metabolism.* Bethesda, MD: Federation of American Societies for Experimental Biology, 1968.

Apseloff, Stanford and Glen Apseloff, M.D. *Executive Diet Helper.* Computer software. Columbus, OH: Ohio Distinctive Software, Inc., 1995.

---. *Food Label Analyzer.* Computer software. Columbus, OH: Ohio Distinctive Software, Inc., 1996.

---. *Menu Planner.* Computer software. Columbus, OH: Ohio Distinctive Software, Inc., 1995.

---. *Weight Loss Planner.* Computer software. Columbus, OH: Ohio Distinctive Software, Inc., 1995.

Beaton, George H. and Earle W. McHenry, eds. *Nutrition.* Vol. 1: *Macronutrients and Nutrient Elements.* New York, NY: Academic Press, 1964.

Food and Nutrition Board Subcommittee on the Tenth Edition of the Recommended Dietary Allowances, Commission on Life Sciences, National Research Council. *Recommended Dietary Allowances.* 10th ed. Washington, DC: National Academy Press, 1989.

Gebhardt, Susan E. and Ruth H. Matthews. *Nutritive Value of Foods.* Revised ed. United States Department of Agriculture. Human Nutrition Information Service. Home and Garden Bulletin 72. Washington, DC: GPO, 1991.

National Cancer Institute Office of Cancer Communications. *Diet, Nutrition & Cancer Prevention: The Good News.* Publication 87-2878. December 1986. Reprinted September 1987.

Nutrition Committee. American Heart Association. *Dietary Guidelines for Healthy American Adults.* 1989.

---. *Exercise and Your Heart.* 1989.

Pollitt, Ernesto and Peggy Amante, eds. *Current Topics in Nutrition and Disease.* Vol. 11: *Energy Intake and Activity*. New York, NY: Alan R. Liss, Inc., 1984.

Powers, Margaret A., MS, RD, CDE, ed. *Nutrition Guide for Professionals. Diabetes Education and Meal Planning.* American Diabetes Association, Inc., and The American Dietetic Association, 1988.

Reed, Patsy B. *Nutrition: An Applied Science.* St. Paul, MN: West Publishing Company, 1980.

Suitor, Carol W. and Merrily F. Hunter. *Nutrition Principles and Application in Health Promotion.* Philadelphia, PA: J.B. Lippincott Company, 1980.

Tver, David F. and Percy Russell, Ph.D. *The Nutrition and Health Encyclopedia.* New York, NY: Van Nostrand Reinhold Company, Inc., 1981.

U.S. Centers for Disease Control and Prevention and American College of Sports Medicine in cooperation with the President's Council on Physical Fitness and Sports. *Summary Statement.* July 1993.

USDA Nutrient Data Base for Standard Reference. March 1984, October 1989, July 1993.

U.S. Department of Agriculture. Nutrition Monitoring Division. Human Nutrition Information Service. *Composition of Foods, 1990 Supplement.* Revised 1991. Washington, DC: GPO, 1991.

Watt, Bernice K. and Annabel L. Merrill. *Composition of Foods.* Agriculture Handbook 8. Consumer and Food Economics Institute. Agricultural Research Service. United States Department of Agriculture. Revised December 1963. Approved for reprinting October 1975. Washington, DC: GPO, 1975.

Whitney, Eleanor N., Corinne B. Cataldo and Sharon R. Rolfes. *Understanding Normal and Clinical Nutrition.* 2nd ed. St. Paul, MN: West Publishing Company, 1987.

Whitney, Eleanor N. and Eva M. N. Hamilton. *Understanding Nutrition.* 4th ed. Revised by Eleanor N. Whitney with Marie A. Boyle. St. Paul, MN: West Publishing Company, 1987.

INDEX

NUTRITION SOFTWARE

PRODUCT INFORMATION AND ORDER FORM

PRODUCTS	PRICE*
Executive Diet Helper – Monitors calories, cholesterol, fat, protein and carbohydrates. Also analyzes and recommends lower-calorie/lower-fat substitute foods. Analyzes individual foods and entire meals from a database of more than 3500 items, including fast foods and frozen dinners.	$4
Menu Planner – Creates daily menu plans for any calorie level and tailors the menus for special needs (e.g., vegetarian, pregnancy, diabetes, hypertension, etc.).	$4
Weight Loss Planner – Recommends calorie consumption based on your physiological profile, determines ideal weight, projects time for weight loss. Analyzes exercises to determine calories burned and weight loss. Provides exercise and diet guidelines. Charts weight loss.	$4
Food Label Analyzer – Analyzes food labels, providing info on calories attributable to fat, protein and carbohydrates, plus info on certain RDA's. Provides tailor-made shoppers' guidelines to ensure foods you buy meet your specifications. Contains an analysis program for foods without labels.	$6

These are exclusive products of Ohio Distinctive Software, Inc., and are not available from any other source. They are all complete programs with instructions and will operate on any PC. **Satisfaction Guaranteed.**

PRODUCT	PRICE*
☐ EXEC DIET HELP	$4
☐ MENU PLANNER	$4
☐ WT LOSS PLAN	$4
☐ FOOD LABEL	$6
Shipping/Handling	+ $3
Total	____

Format:
DOS: ☐5.25" disk ☐3.5" disk
Mac: ☐CD-ROM ☐3.5" disk
Win: ☐CD-ROM ☐3.5" disk

Name______________________

Address______________________

____

***Note**: Please order soon because prices are subject to change without notice. Ohio residents please add 5.75% sales tax. Send this form with payment to: Ohio Distinctive Software, Inc. • 4588 Kenny Road • Columbus OH 43220.